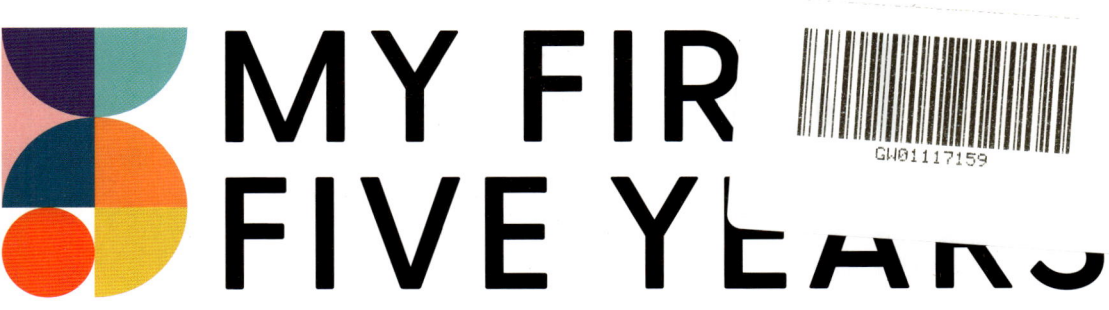

MY FIRST FIVE YEARS

Toddler

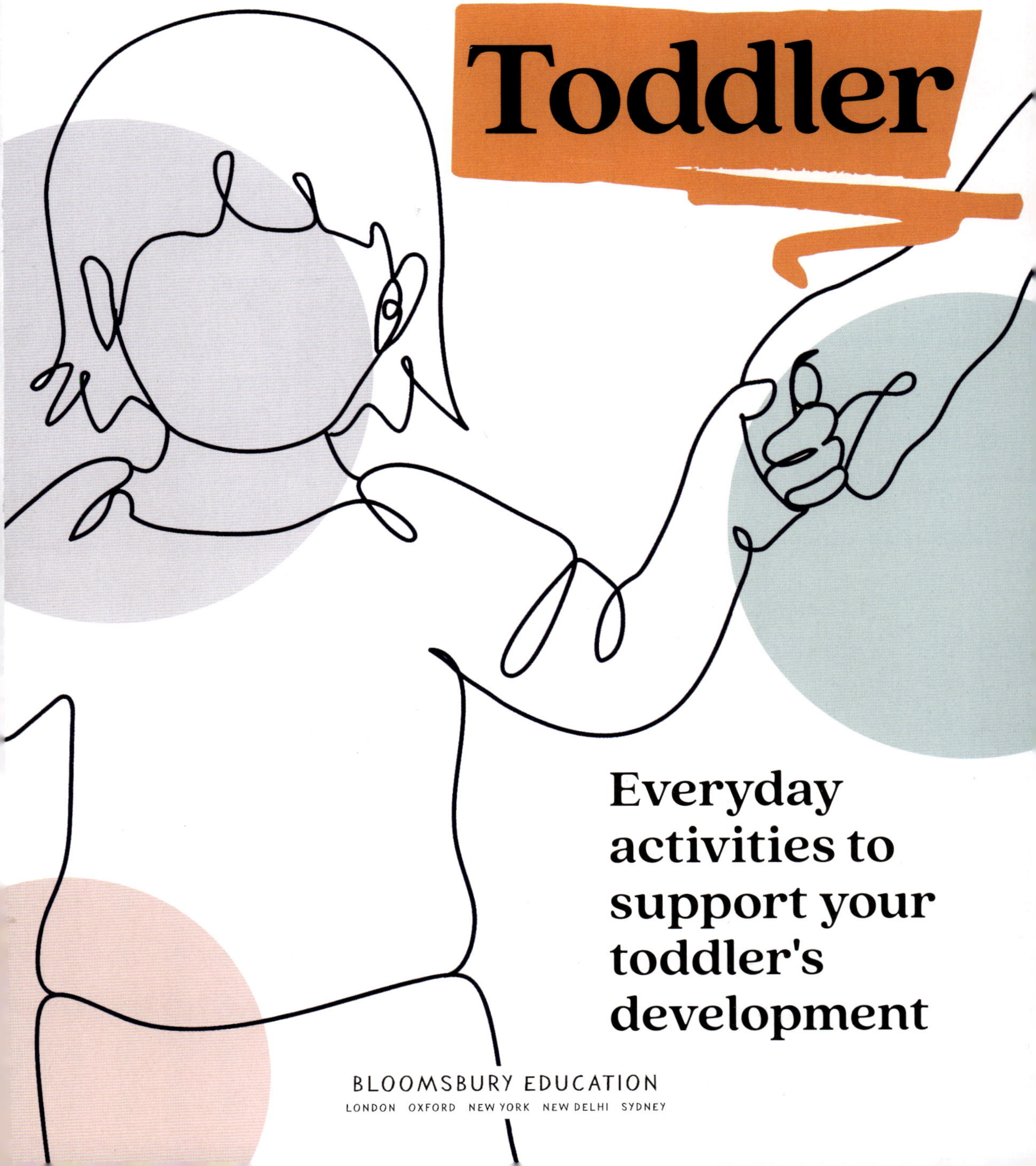

Everyday activities to support your toddler's development

BLOOMSBURY EDUCATION
LONDON OXFORD NEW YORK NEW DELHI SYDNEY

BLOOMSBURY EDUCATION
Bloomsbury Publishing Plc
50 Bedford Square, London, WC1B 3DP, UK
29 Earlsfort Terrace, Dublin 2, Ireland

BLOOMSBURY, BLOOMSBURY EDUCATION and the Diana logo
are trademarks of Bloomsbury Publishing Plc

First published in Great Britain, 2024 by Bloomsbury Publishing Plc
Text copyright © My First Five Years, 2024
Illustrations copyright © My First Five Years, 2024

My First Five Years have asserted their right under the Copyright, Designs and Patents Act, 1988,
to be identified as Author of this work

Bloomsbury Publishing Plc does not have any control over, or responsibility for, any third-party
websites referred to or in this book. All internet addresses given in this book were correct at the time
of going to press. The author and publisher regret any inconvenience caused if addresses have
changed or sites have ceased to exist, but can accept no responsibility for any such changes

All rights reserved. No part of this publication may be reproduced or transmitted in any form or by any
means, electronic or mechanical, including photocopying, recording, or any information storage or
retrieval system, without prior permission in writing from the publishers

A catalogue record for this book is available from the British Library

ISBN: PB: 978-1-8019-9152-0; ePDF: 978-1-8019-9153-7; ePub: 978-1-8019-9154-4

2 4 6 8 10 9 7 5 3 1 (paperback)

Text design by Peter Clayman

Printed and bound in India by Replika Press Pvt. Ltd

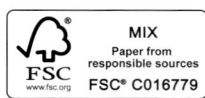

To find out more about our authors and books visit www.bloomsbury.com
and sign up for our newsletters

Acknowledgements
Thank you to Anne Statham, it was your knowledge and passion that
enabled this book to come alive, and to Jennifer Garrity for your beautiful
illustrations and creative vision. Also, to the whole My First Five Years Child
Development Team for their enthusiasm, ideas and support.

Introduction............ 6

The My First Five Years Approach............ 8

How to use this book............ 10

Chapter 1: Social and emotional............ 13
- A family book — The people who are special to me............ 17
- Breakfast in bed — A treat for a special person............ 18
- Dressing up — Who will you be today?............ 19
- Pizza portraits — Edible art............ 20
- Separation ceremonies — Begin to develop a 'goodbye' routine............ 21
- We are all storytellers — Telling your own bedtime tales............ 22
- Bath time play — Give your doll or toy a wash............ 23
- A cosy place — A space to feel safe and calm............ 24
- This one's for you — A moment of self-care............ 25
- What's happening today? — Talking through what to expect............ 26

Chapter 2: Gross motor............ 27
- Hide and seek — An obstacle treasure hunt............ 31
- Twirling ribbon wands — Make some magic as you move............ 32
- DIY window paint — Washable art 33
- Swing ball challenge — Hit the ball as it moves............ 34
- Den making — Can you find your way in?............ 35
- Catch my tail — Running, chasing and dodging!............ 36
- Washing day — Your own cleaning station............ 37
- Peg up the clothes — Laundry time............ 38
- Ladder play — Step, jump and hop!............ 39
- Who threw that? — Play catch like wild animals............ 40

Chapter 3: Fine motor............ 41
- Stone cairns — An ancient tradition to mark a special place............ 44
- Threading tubes — Recycling hack!............ 45
- Cutting tray — Snip it up!............ 46
- Sand stories — Drawing in the ground............ 47
- Whittling away — Safe knife skills............ 48
- Taste-safe paint — Squeezy bottle painting............ 49
- Dough play — Workout for the wrists, hands and fingers............ 50
- Match of the day — Blow football............ 51
- Scoop and splash — Filling, pouring and transferring water............ 52
- Hammering — Real-life skills............ 53

Chapter 4: Sensory............ 54

- Make some whizzy noise — A cardboard tube kazoo............ 59
- Musical statues and bumps — Freeze when the music stops!............ 60
- Roll me, watch me, stop me — Catch the chaos............ 61
- Whisk it up — Bubble beards and wigs............ 62
- Squeezy sensory dough — Play dough with a twist............ 63
- Whose voice is that? — Storytime with family and friends............ 64
- Light and dark — Playing with shadows............ 65
- Skewers for chewers — A taste sensation............ 66
- Hubble bubble toil and trouble — A simple and mobile potion kit............ 67
- Indoor obstacle course — Physical fun with furniture............ 68

Chapter 5: Language............ 69

- Shh! What can you hear? — A listening moment............ 73
- What can it be? — Describing and recognising toys............ 74
- Let's get ready to go — Getting dressed............ 75
- Open all hours — Setting up shop............ 76
- Library time — Sharing stories............ 77
- Ready, steady, go! — Traffic light game............ 78
- A trip to an unfamiliar shop — Exploring somewhere new............ 79
- Tell me more — Talking about experiences............80
- Feeling the beat — Moving to the rhythm............ 81
- Tall tales — Making up stories............ 82

Chapter 6: Cognitive............ 83

- Make a favourite sandwich — Tell others how to do it!............ 87
- I wonder what might happen next — Anticipating events in familiar stories............ 88
- What's missing? — A memory game............ 89
- Recreate a familiar place — Open-ended role play............ 90
- Brick play — Stacking, bridging, enclosing and representing............ 91
- An amazing soundscape — Make your own musical story............ 92
- Full to the top — Exploring capacity in the bath............ 93
- A pictorial calendar — What's happening this week?............ 94
- Let's go shopping — Noticing signs and logos............ 95
- Mix and match — Can you find the other sock?............ 96

> **Play is the super power we all possess!**

Alistair Bryce-Clegg,
My First Five Years Founder

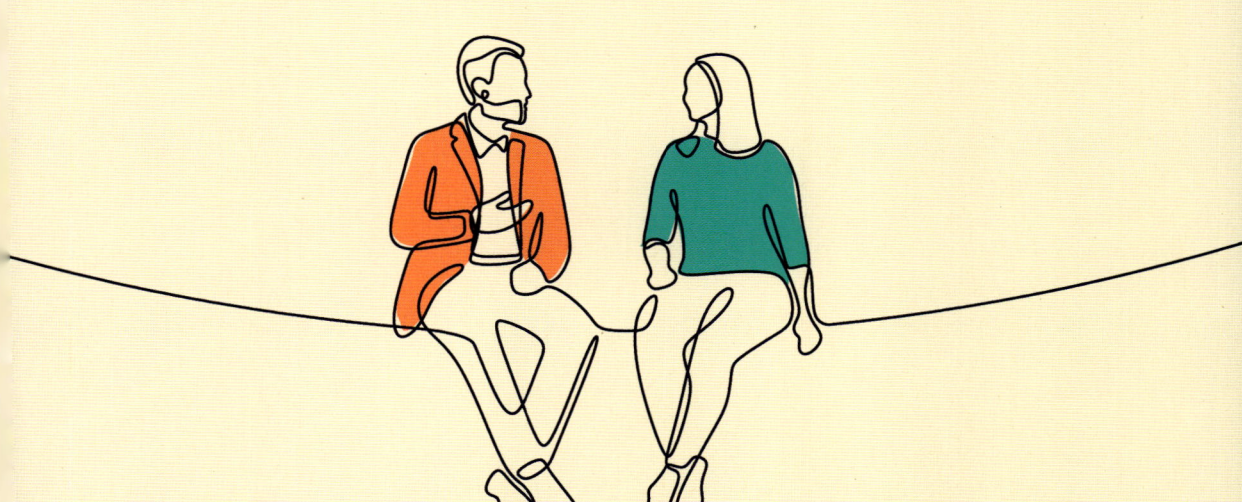

Introduction

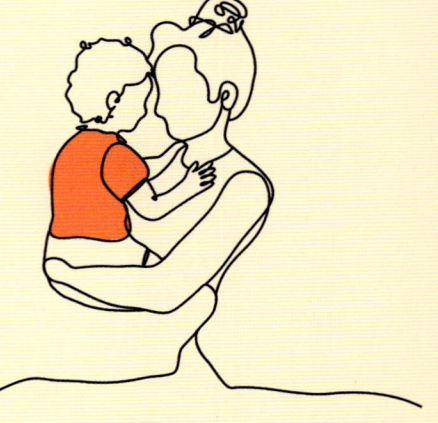

There are days, we are sure, when you are the parent who places a range of colourful, healthy snacks in your toddler's lunchbox, who calmly produces a fresh set of clothes after a mishap, and who has time to stop and admire the smallest creature on the path. We also know that there are plenty of other times when you wonder if, as a parent, you are doing 'enough'.

Yes, spending time with a toddler is like being given the amazing opportunity to explore and discover how awesome the world is all over again. Things you may have disregarded for many years are elevated in importance; the slow-moving hairy caterpillar or the (it turns out, super-friendly) person tipping the rubble from the dumper truck.

It's great to share this wonder with your child, however, other parts of your life continue in the usual way and, for many, return alongside the parenting. Perhaps you are heading back to work and also have other children to care for, resulting in days when caring for your toddler seems never-ending because there are so many other tasks to be done, and the only 'wonder' around is how to juggle everything.

Your toddler needs you, and we are here to support you.

We get this reality. We have thought about how our activities can accompany you through the different times and moods of the parenting journey.

This book will spark your curiosity about the development behind your toddler's intriguing behaviours, philosophical questions and boundless curiosity whilst linking these to the joy of everyday discovery. And the activities will highlight how familiar situations and daily routines (even in those, seemingly, never-ending days) are rich in possibilities for playing, chatting, responding, cuddling and even relaxing.

We know that comparing your child's pace of development to others is often a source of worry. Our activities give your toddler time to explore, revisit and connect learning experiences at their own pace as we encourage you to take the parenting scenic route and notice the beautiful moments along the way. Whether you are a brand new or more experienced parent, you can feel comforted by discovering how the small magical daily moments you share together are so important, and how simple adjustments and enhancements can maximise these moments.

We use the term toddler throughout our book but purposefully do not link this to a specific age, rather we think of toddlerhood beginning the moment that your child pulls themselves to standing and takes their first steps. Other significant changes in development we describe follow a typical pattern but can occur over a wide timescale.

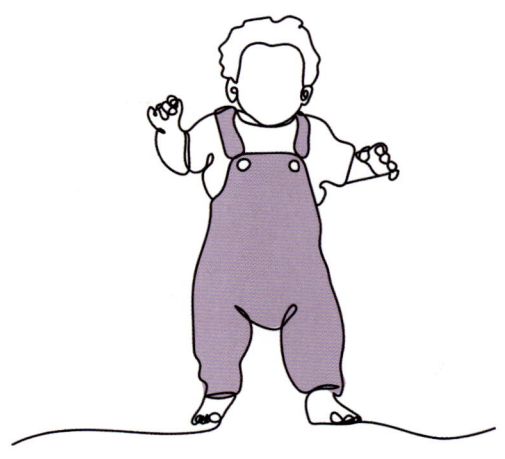

The essence of being a toddler is about the big changes in brain development, growing more of a sense of being an individual, using language to communicate and think and of course having the physical ability to move with more independence and control.

Toddlerhood does not occur in isolation; all that has gone before has brought your child to this moment, and you know their unique story so far. This personal story gives you the backdrop to their thinking and unique view of the world and we encourage you to keep this context in mind as you dip in and select the activities that you know will suit your child best.

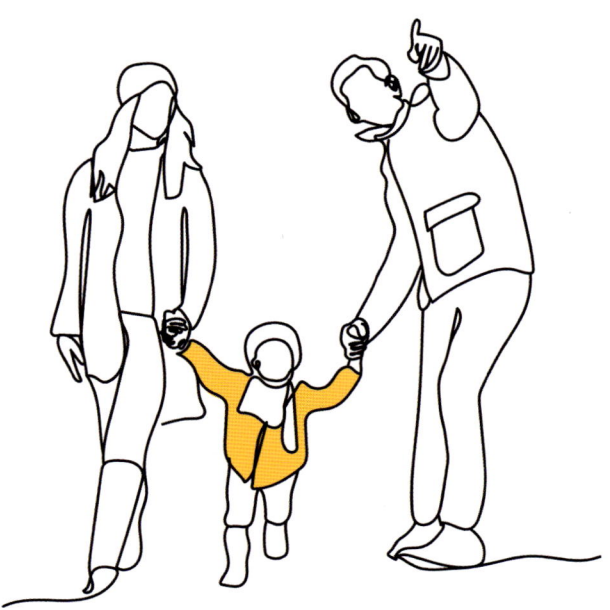

The My First Five Years approach

It's all about play!

We at My First Five Years like to shout loudly about the importance of play! Our firm belief is that play is definitely not the opposite of work. Play certainly isn't always just for fun – play can be a serious thing for a toddler. It can be scientific, mathematical, creative, and involves testing ideas, making connections, adapting approaches, persevering and much more.

Concerns about 'hitting milestones' and achieving goals within certain timescales can lead to more formal and adult-directed learning approaches which tend to hurry children, even toddlers, through structured experiences, squeezing time for play, especially free play, out of their lives at a very early age.

We want to reset the balance.

We know that play can be so many things, and its importance cannot be underestimated. Lots of words can be used to describe play, such as wondrous, challenging, absorbing, exploratory, caring, evolving, quiet, boisterous, social, creative, imaginative, skilful, emotional... the list could go on forever!

Watching your toddler will show you that their drive to play is natural and irrepressible and bubbles to the surface in the most unlikely, and least obviously playful, situations! At this time, your toddler's curiosity and need to actively explore will be at an all-time high, and they now have the growing independence to widen their explorations and experience of the world as they set off on their own two feet – probably with you in hot pursuit!

You might find that your toddler loves being outside; many of our activities give them this option. Playing outdoors is not only essential for your toddler to understand, value, enjoy and protect our natural world, it gives them a treasure trove of unique experiences and play opportunities.

> **Playing is central to children's spontaneous drive for development, and it performs a significant role in the development of the brain, particularly in the early years.**
>
> United Nations Convention on the Rights of the Child[1]

[1] Committee on the Rights of the Child (2013) General comment No. 17 on the rights of the child to rest, leisure, play, recreational activities, cultural life and the arts (art. 31). Conventions on the Rights of the child: United Nations.

Knowledge is power!
We know you are, absolutely, the expert when it comes to your toddler, but sometimes you might want to know a bit more about the science behind their development. Our activity ideas are underpinned by knowledge and research, and we give simple pointers to interesting and relevant facts about toddler development so you can feel empowered to make informed choices.

Relationships are at the heart of all learning
We are sure you know that all the best learning happens in a playful, relaxed way as your toddler interacts with you or other people who are important to them. Family life and rich relationships are part of learning, so we have included activity ideas that can become a playful part of your whole family's regular routine.

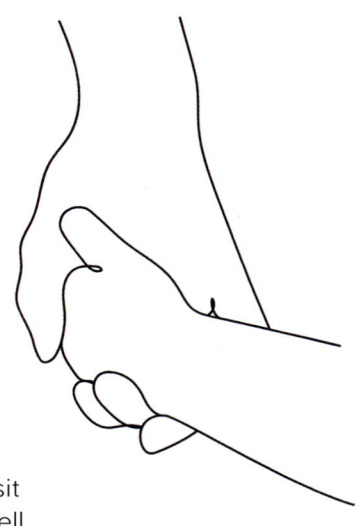

Again, again and again
Repetition is an important part of learning as it supports deeper thinking through giving your toddler the opportunity to revisit, connect and consolidate skills. We love the idea of wallowing in learning! We encourage you and your toddler to take it slowly and revisit activities again and again, in order to learn deeply and well.

It's important for your toddler to enjoy the feeling of mastery involved in doing something they have done before they perhaps take it a little step further. You can take time to notice and build up skills at the pace that is right for your toddler.

A realistic approach
Our realistic parenting approach means you won't find Instagram-style ideas (which take hours to set up) in our books. Instead, we offer ideas and activities that you can fit into everyday life which are relevant and meaningful to you and your toddler.

Learning happens in lots of incidental ways and we highlight opportunities for you to support your toddler's learning through moments in your daily routine, such as getting dressed, preparing meals or going on a journey.

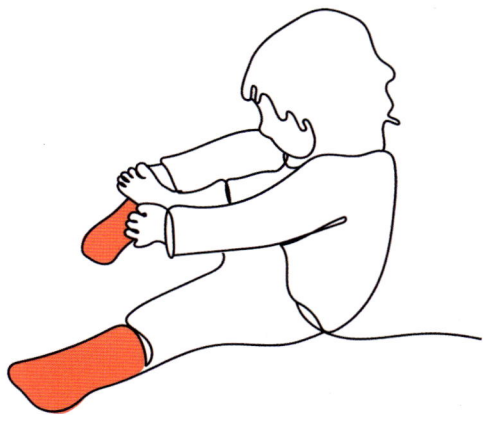

When you are depleted, it can be helpful to focus on some caregiving activities and give them your full attention, including cuddles, chatting face to face and responding to your toddler's gentle cues for interaction. Take these activities slowly and they can bolster your own emotional reserves, as well as your toddler's.

It is important to recognise how you are feeling and know that having a hard day or feeling anxious or upset can be part of parenting. If these feelings feel too difficult to cope with alone, or if you feel like this a lot of the time, speak to a health professional or someone you trust. You can also contact charities, like PANDAS, who support parents.

How to use this book

Introduction to our six streams of development

At My First Five Years, we use six streams of development to describe children's learning and development.

- Social and emotional
- Gross motor
- Fine motor
- Sensory
- Language
- Cognitive

Like a stream, your toddler will carve out a learning journey that will sometimes meander gently, sometimes race ahead like rapids and sometimes be still for a time before moving on. Although your toddler's development may look similar to others it is totally unique, as the journey of no two children, or streams, is ever the same.

The six chapters in this book are organised around these six streams of development. Each chapter outlines and explains developmental highlights within a particular stream of development for your toddler and offers you ten playful activity ideas to try together.

There is no need to work through a particular section from beginning to end; the streams interweave so you can dip in anywhere and try an activity you think your toddler will enjoy.

Thinking about learning in terms of these streams can help you to notice the small steps your toddler takes before they reach particular milestones. We think marveling in all of these small moments, as well as the bigger milestones, will help you to find the joy in parenting!

Equipment

Our activities make use of recycled items, household objects and natural materials, rather than requiring special equipment or costly resources. We anticipate that you can find these items at your fingertips ready to go, although you may not have thought of them as 'toys' or learning resources before!

The variety of colours, shapes, weights, sizes, materials and textures of many everyday items are intriguing to your toddler and this encourages them to investigate more closely by handling them, exploring them with all their senses and using their imagination to discover more about what each item is like, what it can do or even what it can become.

Active play

We focus on activities that allow your toddler to move and explore freely and use their whole body as we know this is how they learn best. We consciously avoid suggesting that your toddler needs to be sat at a table or contained in a chair to participate. You will notice that many activities also suggest that, if possible, you join your toddler in their play, sharing their level and perspective on the floor.

Food play

We feel strongly that food should not be wasted, but we also know that food play offers lots of valuable sensory experiences for toddlers and can be especially useful for younger children who are still exploring the world using their mouths.

Experiencing food through play can give your toddler the confidence to try eating a wide variety of foods as they grow. Using some edible items in play gives your toddler freedom to explore the taste, texture, smell and look of foods without the pressure to eat them which comes at mealtimes.

For this reason, we have chosen to retain some food products in our activities, however, we have made several decisions to help reduce waste. We anticipate that the food chosen is a type that can be reused many times and, where we can, we offer alternatives to a food product. Some of our ideas, such as home-made play dough, can't avoid using food-based ingredients (in this case flour) so we would encourage you to keep your dough once you finish an activity so that you can reuse it many times.

The activities

Each activity is organised in the same way:

What you need lists the resources needed for each activity.

The steps gives you step-by-step instructions for carrying out the activity.

Benefits for your toddler highlights the skills your toddler will be developing from the activity.

Building on gives you ideas for adapting the activity to suit you and your toddler.

Routine hack
Some activities encourage you to tweak your usual daily routine, just a little, to maximise the learning possibilities of incidental moments, such as whilst your toddler is getting dressed, preparing meals together or bath times. These activities are identified by our Routine hack symbol.

Safety
Some activities have Safety notices; these indicate extra precautions you might take or things to consider.

QR code
Find out more about how My First Five Years provides you with tools, knowledge and support to block out unhelpful comparisons, feel more confident and better understand the way in which your toddler learns and develops.

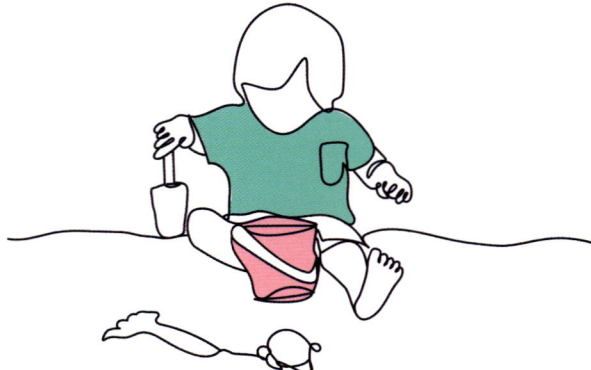

Chapter 1

Social and emotional

Finding out about myself, making relationships and gaining a sense of belonging!

Being social is very complicated! Happily, your toddler is wired for social connection and they will be developing their sense of identity and belonging through tuning into the safe, strong network of relationships that surrounds them.

You and other close familiar adults create a safe haven from which your toddler can explore, giving them a strong foundation on which to develop the confidence to venture further, take a few calculated risks and test out new things, safe in the knowledge that there is a secure place to return to for reassurance and help if needed. Although it feels a long way off, this will eventually be the same launch pad from which they set out independently into the world.

Your toddler will be watching and picking up cues all of the time from their close relationships and even from encounters with strangers. They will watch carefully and assess how you and others react and respond to them, to other people and to different situations.

In a similar way to forming attachments with people, your toddler may show attachment to familiar and well-loved places or items, such as a favourite toy, a soft blanket or a special space. Understandably, they might find it hard to separate or share these, just as we adults find it difficult to share a favourite chair, a usual spot around a meeting table, a well-loved cup or a treasured old pair of socks! Special objects are sometimes referred to as 'comforters' or 'transitional objects'. These constant and familiar items have an important role as they travel with your toddler (or you) and bring comfort in different or new places.

Your toddler will be becoming more aware of the wide range of different feelings and emotions – some positive and some negative – they are experiencing. These feelings and emotions translate as physical sensations and their body might feel a bit scarily out of control or dysregulated. For example, when they are tired or fearful, their heartbeat will rise to prepare for a fight or flight response.

Toddlers will use their behaviour as a means of communicating their need for connection, reassurance, protection and support, as they haven't yet got adequate words to explain these feelings. In fact, even as adults, understanding and explaining our feelings is often still a work in progress. As a parent, it can be an emotionally challenging time for you too, as your toddler looks to you to help them regulate these sometimes-overwhelming feelings and emotions and to help to return them to a calm baseline.

Each time you co-regulate alongside your toddler, with your warm responsive interaction during times of distress, upset or difficulty, you demonstrate strategies to help them to understand, express or regulate their thoughts and feelings. These might be the times when you help your toddler to calm down through a soothing cuddle or by modelling deep breaths, when you hold their hand and give it a squeeze, when you support them to try to put their feelings into words or when you help them to reason through a tricky situation and plan what to do to navigate a difficulty.

This co-regulation through experience is really important as it provides your toddler with a sort of 'blueprint' to manage triggers; a concrete understanding or selection of strategies to draw on to help with handling overwhelming emotions. If provided consistently, it will help them to navigate emotional and physical discomfort and eventually to learn to be able to soothe themselves or self-regulate and hence bounce back with resilience.

Your toddler will also begin to recognise that feelings are not only personal to them but shared by others too. This is sometimes called developing 'theory of mind' which is how one person develops an internal conception of the emotional state of others.

Your toddler may begin to seek closeness and become a friend to others as their understanding of their own feelings and emotions develops. Understanding their own emotions is the first step in allowing your toddler to begin to have concern and empathy for the feelings of others.

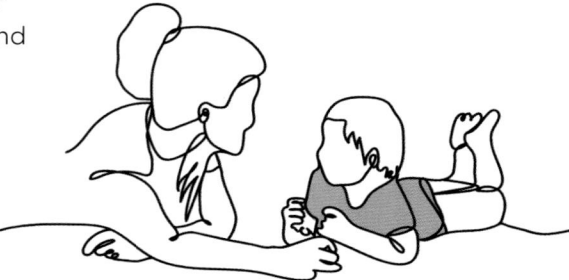

As your toddler begins to show interest in other children, they might test out strategies to join in play or work out how they can have a turn with a popular toy. There might be times when they try to achieve their goal through a range of different behaviours. For example, they might chase other children to join play or other children might chase them, or they may come close to others by playing alongside them and mirroring the play. They may even seek connection by taking the toy another child is playing with to see what happens! Your toddler's developing language skills are also useful for building these social connections as they begin to share their thoughts, opinions and ideas.

Self-confidence and self-awareness will be growing stronger as the front part of your toddler's brain, the prefrontal cortex, develops. This development continues into adulthood, so really this is just the very beginning of the journey. Your toddler will develop the skills to plan, organise and predict outcomes as their experience of the world and associated memory bank grows. Self-confidence will allow your toddler to be secure in their own opinions and to realise that these are important although separate to the opinions of others who might have differing ideas.

> **As well as reaching into our own minds we reach into the minds of others.**
>
> Maria Robinson[1]

The activities in this book support your toddler to explore some of these complex skills safely and playfully, by watching and listening to what is going on around them, exploring the nature of different relationships, having their feelings and opinions listened to and affirmed, and by being encouraged to express themselves in their own unique way.

Building relationships

Your toddler's view of the world is shaped by the relationships they have with you, your family, friends and other adults they see frequently, perhaps in the wider community. These close relationships give your toddler an understanding of how warm, loving and nurturing relationships work, along with a sense of belonging and safety.

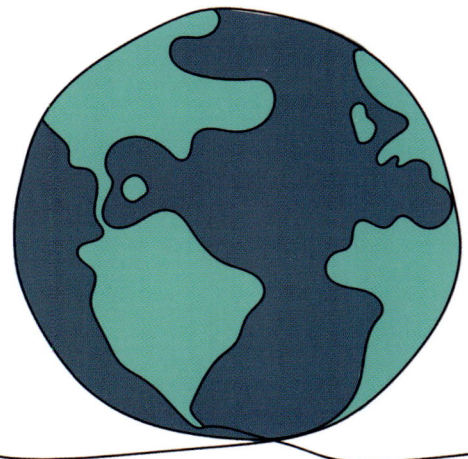

Developing a sense of self and belonging
Your toddler will be exploring their identity by noticing and perhaps pointing out ways they are similar to or different from others. This may be related to aspects of physical appearance or their preferences and opinions.

Your toddler may declare how their view is different to yours and may enjoy discovering the power of 'no'! Although this may feel tricky to navigate, it is an important part of your toddler knowing themselves and their mind. These feelings of identity can be supported as you make attempts to understand what your child is thinking and explore this through giving simple choices where possible. The more you tune into your toddler and help them to express themselves in words, the more understood they will feel.

Developing a sense of independence
As the sense of being a unique individual develops, your toddler will be keen to do more things for themselves, such as day-to-day tasks or care routines, and with this a growing sense of autonomy will develop.

Understanding, expressing and regulating emotions
As your child becomes a toddler, they will experience a wider range of more complex emotions which might sometimes overwhelm them. They will be testing out ways to express, understand and process these emotions. Experience with emotions informs understanding; by repeating experiences or thinking back or reflecting on situations and the associated feelings and emotions, your toddler can understand them better.

They will learn how adults respond to their expressions of emotion. For example, your angry toddler needs to feel understood even if their accompanying behaviour is to be discouraged. You can help your toddler by continuing to provide consistent responses to their feelings and emotions through co-regulation.

Self-regulation ultimately grows from this basis and could be described as the ability to adapt behaviour to the circumstances, according to your own set of internal rules, rather than reacting to the situation. As your toddler recognises their feelings are not only personal to them but shared by others too, they will become able to empathise with others.

QR code
Don't forget to scan this QR code to find lots more child development content and bonus activity ideas from the team at My First Five Years.

[1] Robinson, M. (2008), *Child Development From Birth to Eight: A Journey Through the Early Years.* Open University Press.

A family book
The people who are special to me

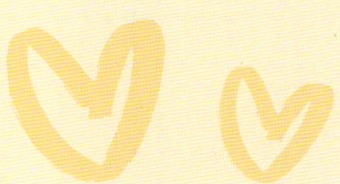

What you need:
- A smart phone or a camera to take photos
- A printer
- A few visits to family or friends' homes
- A blank book and a glue stick

The steps:
- When you visit a family member or friend, take a camera with you.
- Take a close-up photo of the important person's face, but also of the things that have a special link to that person. So, for example, this might be their front door, their pet, their lounge or kitchen, their car, their hobbies or their garden.
- Encourage your toddler to be involved in choosing what to photograph; you will know what interests them most when they visit.
- Print out the photos and make them into a family book that you can look at and talk about together.

Benefits for your toddler:
- Being reminded of their close relationships through looking at the book gives your toddler a sense of belonging and safety.
- Supports your toddler to reflect on their identity by noticing and perhaps pointing out the ways in which they are like, or different from, others. This may be related to aspects of their physical appearance, the type of home they live in or the things they prefer to do.

Building on:
- Add to this book over time and allow your toddler to take some of the photos themselves.
- Note down what your toddler says about the photos to add some text to the book.
- You could display photos in a 'family tree' showing relationships between people – for example, siblings, parents, grandparents, cousins and so on.

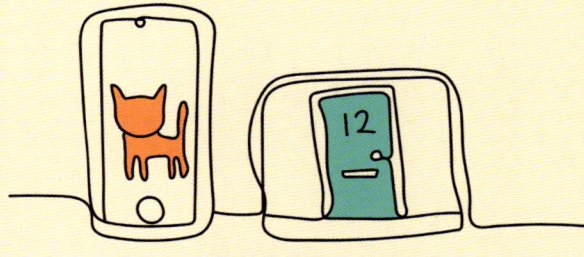

Breakfast in bed
A treat for a special person

What you need:

- Breakfast food items
- Bowls, plates and cutlery
- A tray
- A few additional special touches, such as a sticky note with a kiss, a flower or a cuddly toy to sit alongside the food
- A recipient for the breakfast (parent, sibling, grandparent or friend)

The steps:

- Explain to your toddler that you are going to make a special breakfast together for a special person or people.
- Help your toddler to get involved in the process as you gather the bowls, plates, cups or utensils you need and place them on the tray, along with the food.
- Talk about what your special person likes for breakfast and how they might feel when you surprise them with breakfast in bed.
- Encourage your toddler to think about what the extra special decoration for the tray might be – they might select a favourite toy, draw a picture or fetch a flower.
- Quietly help your toddler to carry the tray and surprise the lucky recipient!

Benefits for your toddler:

- Doing something kind for someone else helps your toddler to develop their sense of empathy as they anticipate and then see the response of others.
- Develops your toddler's growing sense of independence and pride in their abilities.
- Develops your toddler's sense of belonging and participation in the family or community.

Building on:

- Your toddler could help you to plan and make other meals for your family and friends – for example, they could make a sandwich with their own special choice of filling.

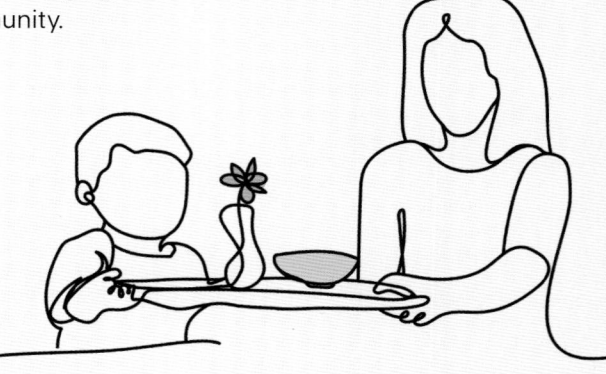

Dressing up
Who will you be today?

What you need:

- A trip to a local charity shop to gather items of different styles and made with different fabrics, such as hats, belts, bags, scarves, jackets and jewellery
- A long mirror
- A bag or box in which to house your dressing up collection

The steps:

- Head out with your toddler to visit some charity shops.
- Keep an open mind about the sorts of outfits you might find; be guided by the things that you see and the possibilities they offer for costumes.
- Avoid 'pre-determined' costumes such as superheroes and princesses. Instead, choose open-ended real-life dressing up clothes that will offer your toddler the opportunity to become different characters.
- Talk to your toddler about the different types of items (hats, dresses, jewellery and so on) and the different types of fabric (leather, denim, cotton and so on). Perhaps link clothing choices to the characters your toddler is familiar with from stories or from real life.
- When you have made your selection, head home to wash or clean any clothes and jewellery as necessary before helping your toddler to try on the items.
- Join in the play with your toddler as their character heads off for an adventure.

Benefits for your toddler:

- Being unrestrained by traditional 'commercialised' play costumes, which dictate a certain type of play, transforms the possibilities of dressing up for your toddler.
- Promotes authentic, real-life and fantasy play, as well as creativity.
- Allows your toddler to explore an infinite range of roles and removes constraints of gender stereotyping.

Building on:

- You could take photos of your toddler in their different costumes.
- Encourage your toddler to give a name to the characters they have created.

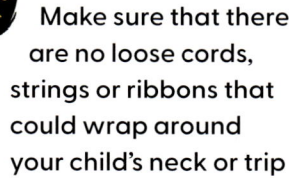

Make sure that there are no loose cords, strings or ribbons that could wrap around your child's neck or trip them (or you) up.

Pizza portraits
Edible art

What you need:
- Pizza bases, either ready-made (fresh or frozen) or home-made
- A tomato-based sauce for the pizza topping
- Cheese or a dairy-free alternative
- Pizza toppings to create features, such as red pepper for the mouth, cucumber and olives for the eyes, grated carrot or broccoli for hair and pepperoni for rosy cheeks
- A selection of small bowls
- A child-safe knife
- A spoon
- Small mirrors to check reflections
- Baking trays
- An oven

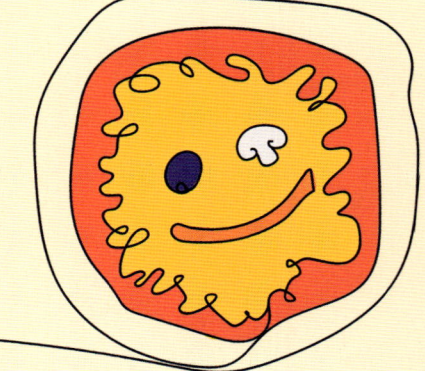

The steps:
- This activity is fun to do with family or friends.
- Your toddler can help you to chop and organise into bowls the different toppings you have chosen for your pizzas.
- Ask your toddler to give each person their pizza base and a mirror to check their reflection.
- Get creative and invite everyone to make a portrait of their face on the pizza base. Talk about your family and friends' different facial features, hair colours and styles, noting similarities and differences as you create the pizzas.
- When the pizzas have been completed, place all of the portrait pizzas together and admire before cooking and eating!

Benefits for your toddler:
- Preparing and sharing food together is a great opportunity to build relationships, chat together and work cooperatively to achieve a goal.
- Your toddler will learn that everyone approaches a task in their own way and creates their pizza with their own unique style.

Building on:
- Your toddler could playfully judge the pizzas with different categories such as tastiness, presentation, likeness to the person and so on.

Separation ceremonies
Begin to develop a 'goodbye' routine

What you need:
- A familiar and trusted adult
- An item that is special to your child

The steps:
- As your toddler grows in independence, the instances where you need to separate from each other, perhaps for daycare or visiting relatives or friends for a time, will become more frequent.
- There is no right or wrong time to begin the process of having some time apart.
- It's helpful to think about these times in advance. If possible, have a few practice runs with a familiar and trusted adult outside of the immediate family. Initially, this can be for a very brief period of time that allows your toddler to understand that when you leave you will always come back.
- Remember that the big emotions of parting are shared by you both. Talk to your child about your own feelings, assuring them that you will miss them whilst you are apart.
- Create your own unique ritual for saying goodbye. You know yourself and your toddler best; you might like a long cuddle, a quick kiss or a pat, or perhaps a high five. If possible, try to pass on confidence to your toddler that they will be OK without you.
- Your toddler might have a favourite toy, comfort blanket or other item that they often seek for reassurance. This object helps your toddler to feel safe and secure, not only because it feels cuddly and nice to touch but also because it offers a sense of continuity between places. Ensure this item forms part of your separation routine.
- You could leave an item of yours also, such as a jumper or bag, to reassure your toddler that you will be back.

Benefits for your toddler:
- We learn to be social through an ever-widening set of relationships. Through spending time with others your toddler can diversify their social world to form a network of supportive emotional bonds (as can you as a parent).

Building on:
- You could talk in simple terms to your toddler about how you missed them when you return, modelling the language of your own feelings and letting them know you were holding them in your mind.

We are all storytellers
Telling your own bedtime tales

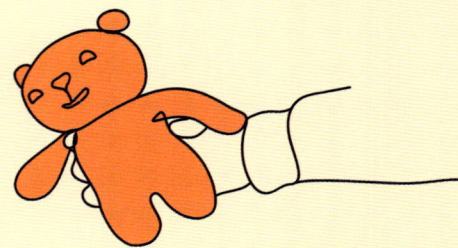

What you need:

- Some of your toddler's favourite toys, such as soft toys, vehicles and play figures – anything goes!
- A range of fabrics and other familiar objects (optional)

The steps:

- Explain to your toddler that you are going to tell a story without a book – it will be a story about their toys.
- Use your imagination to make up your story; think about where the story is set, who the main characters are (you could include yourself or your toddler as characters) and perhaps a problem they encounter and need to solve.
- Pause in your storytelling and leave space and time for your toddler to contribute their ideas, perhaps by saying, 'I wonder what happened after that… let me think…'.
- You can use experiences and feelings that your child has encountered to shape your story. For example, if they have been sad because they fell over, your character could have the same experience and talk about their feelings. Alternatively, if your child has been worried about the dark, your story could explore these fears and offer solutions.
- With practice, telling your own story becomes easier and your toddler will be confident to join in more. Your stories could weave together and build on the ones you have told before.

Benefits for your toddler:

- Making up personal stories whilst safely snuggling together allows your toddler to reflect on and express emotions and feeling about situations they have encountered.
- They can learn that emotions and feelings are shared and can explore possible solutions to situations they are finding tricky.

Building on:

- Retell favourite stories and allow your toddler to prompt you to remember the sequence of events and what happened next.

Bath time play
Give your doll or toy a wash

What you need:

- A washing up bowl, large plastic container or baby bath
- A doll or toy figure in need of a wash
- Bubble bath and a flannel

The steps:

- Explain to your toddler that their doll or toy figure is going to have a bath. Follow the same routine you usually follow together when your toddler has their bath.
- Use plenty of words to describe what's going on as your toddler washes the doll or toy, naming parts of the body and actions such as 'wash', 'splash' and 'dry'.
- Give your toddler simple instructions like, 'Shall we wash baby's hair?'.
- When bath time is finished, dry the doll or toy and dress if necessary.

Benefits for your toddler:

- We know that it's important for all children to experience play that involves care routines because it supports growing empathy.
- Running though familiar daily routines playfully helps your toddler to understand the steps of their own daily routines and anticipate what happens next. It's useful for parts of the routine they may not usually look forward to.
- Talking through routines allows your toddler to link language related to routine, which can additionally help them to emotionally process events.
- It's a chance to revisit things they've heard from adults by playing the adult role themselves. You might notice your toddler acting out instructions and things you've said to them.
- This imaginative role play is helping your toddler develop their social skills as they explore a familiar situation from a different perspective – seeing what things are like for others.

Building on:

- Role play other parts of your toddler's routine together; perhaps pretend to clean the doll or toy's teeth for two minutes, or put the doll or toy to bed.

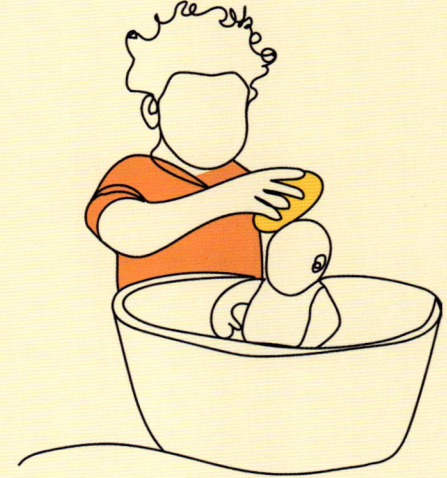

A cosy place
A space to feel safe and calm

What you need:

- A small space in your home that your toddler can feel belongs to them, such as a corner of their bedroom, a space in the lounge or a small area behind furniture
- Soft furnishings, such as fabrics, cushions, pillows and blankets
- Clothes pegs
- A selection of soft toys and books

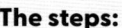

The steps:

- Your toddler might have already shown you the special places in your home where they like to play. These are often small nooks or corners where your toddler feels safe, cosy and secure in their own private space.
- Encourage your toddler to enhance a space with you. Offer them the selection of soft furnishings and let them take the lead in organising the area. You could make a roof using the fabric and pegs or create a place for the toys to sit.
- When the den is created, your child might want to invite you in – or they might prefer to keep you out! They may want to read a story with you or engage in role play.
- If possible, keep the cosy den in place for a while and watch how your toddler's play evolves.

Benefits for your toddler:

- The secret space gives your toddler privacy. Through having their own hideaway place to create in their style and to go to unaccompanied, they are beginning to create their own rules and sense of individual identity in a secure environment.
- Over time, your toddler might use the space to help them to begin to regulate their emotions; a place to go to help them calm down and reset.
- Spending time together with your toddler in their 'home from home' builds a warm relationship where you are following your toddler's rules, for a change!

Building on:

- You could make a sign for the cosy den with your child's name on it to enhance the sense it belongs to them.
- The space is a great area for your toddler to share if friends come around to play.

This one's for you
A moment of self-care

What you need:

- Some time at the end of a busy day

The steps:

- Think about things that have happened during the day with your toddler that you have enjoyed or are proud of. Perhaps you managed to support a tricky behaviour or helped with a strong emotion, or maybe your toddler showed you some new learning or something that made you laugh.

- Choose three things and give yourself a pat on the back!

- If you find you have worries and concerns that come to mind, consider how you could voice those and to whom you could speak, such as a partner, family member or friend. Talking through a problem can have positive results and asking for help is a good thing.

Benefits for your toddler:

- Taking care of a toddler can be challenging and exhausting and it can raise strong feelings and emotions. If you have the opportunity to rest, recharge and feel good, there is a better chance your toddler will feel good too!

- Your wellbeing and your toddler's wellbeing intertwine.

Building on:

- Perhaps build a habit of writing down the three positive things each day. You can read back through these at difficult moments or keep them as a memento for when your toddler is older.

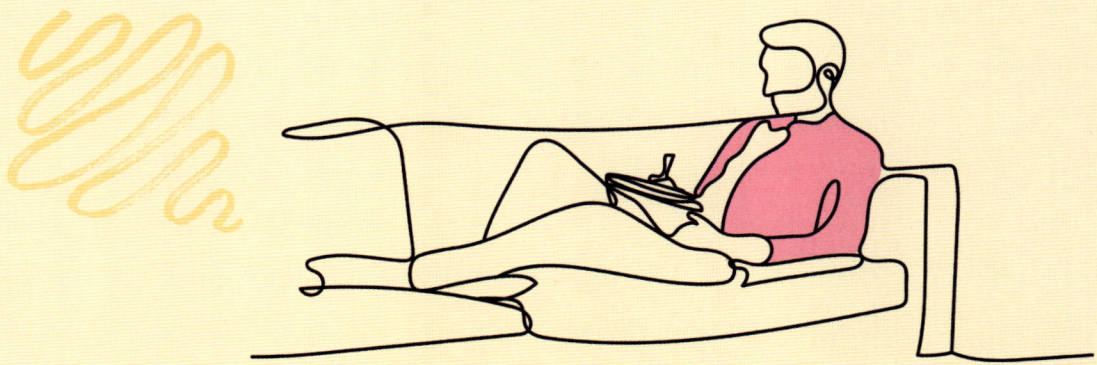

What's happening today?
Talking through what to expect

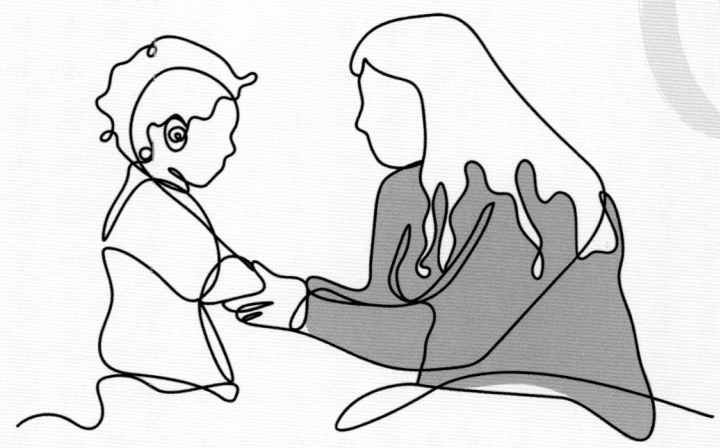

What you need:

No equipment needed

The steps:

- In the morning, talk through with your toddler the main events of your day. This might begin with a simple 'now and next' conversation. For example, 'Now we are eating breakfast, next we will walk to the park'.
- As your toddler's understanding grows, you can sequence more of the day's upcoming events for them. For example, 'After breakfast we will walk to the park. When we leave the park, we will pop into the shop to buy something for lunch'.

Benefits for your toddler:

- Helping children to anticipate what is going to happen during the day gives their day some structure which can alleviate anxiety.
- This understanding enables them to feel secure in the day's routine just as we, as adults, like to anticipate what might happen to us in a new situation.
- Talking through situations in advance gives your toddler the chance to express and resolve with you any worries they might have.

Building on:

- Talking through daily events in advance gives your child the chance to be involved in shaping the day, including opportunities for them to make choices about what to do, where to go and how long to stay.

Chapter 2

Gross motor

Get moving!

As the parent of a toddler, you are probably witnessing first-hand that it is natural for your child to be engaged in almost constant movement! This wonderful energy comes as the part of your toddler's brain involved in the regulation and control of movement is maturing quickly.

Cleverly, your toddler's body is naturally driven to get what it needs from, and to interact with, the environment around them. So, a low wall invites them to balance along it; a tree with low-hanging branches (or an adult's body) prompts them to climb or hang off it; a large open field invites them to run and so on. These aren't conscious decisions – they are instincts that your toddler has because they must run and climb and spin and roll to grow the body systems they need for life.

Movement and early learning intertwine; cognitive areas of the brain are being fired up as different ways to move are tested and repeated. Your toddler will be creating an internal three-dimensional map of space, considering how to plan their movements and judge time and speed, both of themselves and other moving things. At first, during the early stages of learning these skills, there will be lots of concentration and brain activity needed but gradually, as the neural pathways are reinforced, your toddler's physical actions will become more automatic. Just like when adults learn a new skill, such as driving a car or hitting a ball with a racquet.

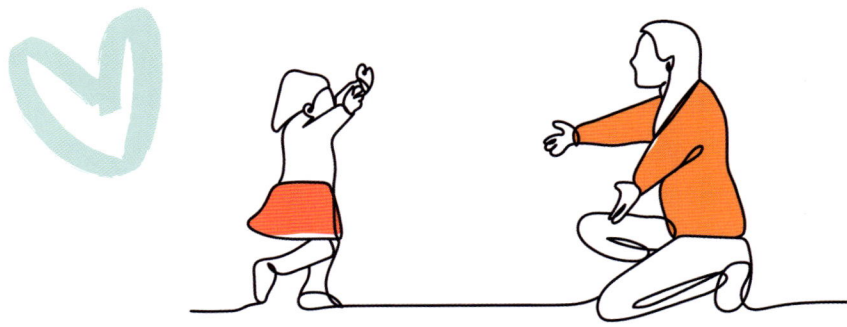

Sometimes it may feel as if there is some conflict between a world built for adults and the small children navigating it. There are social expectations, sometimes even rules, around how we should use our body and move through public spaces. Children want and need to be on the move but might find themselves in situations where they are told by adults to 'Stand still' or are only praised for restraining movement, for 'Lovely sitting still', and so on, making your toddler think they need to ignore their desire to move.

In contrast, the activities in this book encourage you to embrace your toddler's inbuilt instinct to move and wriggle rather than suggesting you try to tame it! Climbing, jumping and spinning allows your toddler to use the stimuli around them to get what their body needs.

Developing postural control and balance

Each movement that your toddler makes when learning to squat, sit, stand, walk, run, balance on one leg, and even throw a ball, will create a shift in their centre of gravity which redistributes the weight of their body. Sudden growth spurts can also cause a shift in your toddler's centre of gravity, meaning they need to make new adjustments to maintain their posture.

Your toddler needs to learn to adjust this centre of gravity as they move, in order to stay balanced or upright – they will learn to manage this process as they embark on a journey of discovery during a variety of daily actions. When your child moves, their brain processes information from their senses. This information helps them to adjust their position and maintain their balance and posture. Lots of practice strengthens these neural connections.

The activities in this book foster creative ways for your toddler to challenge their balance in relation to different ways of moving. We explore spinning, turning or rolling movements, back and forth movements like swinging or rocking, and up and down movements like jumping or bouncing. Do not worry when your toddler falls over as falling is an important part of learning!

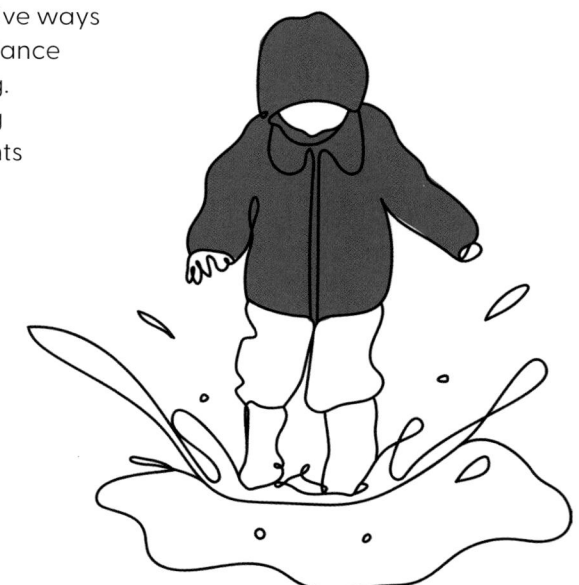

These gross motor activities also link to those in our sensory development chapter which challenge our vestibular system and also help us understand our movement and position.

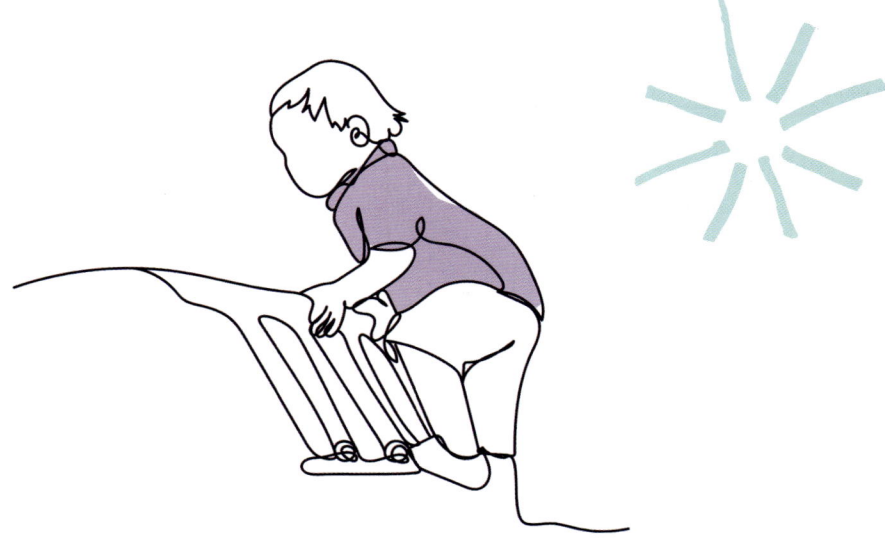

Strengthening upper body and core muscles
When we talk about your toddler's 'core' we are referring to the set of muscles that are located at the centre of their body. These core muscles help them to generate the power to move. Core muscles also stabilise the body and provide a solid base of support from which your toddler's arms and legs are free to move with precision and control.

As your toddler's core muscles developed, they will have firstly explored how to stand, using their arms to pull themselves up. As they grew stronger they would have learnt to cruise, moving around in a standing position while holding onto furniture. These skills will have helped them to develop their balance, and now that their body is able to stand in a stable, upright position without support, they are able to distribute their weight as they step.

Gross motor skills form the foundation upon which subsequent fine motor development takes place. This core balance allows your toddler's shoulders, arms, elbows, wrists and hands to move freely, allowing them to perform a new range of large motor movements.

Shoulder, elbow and wrist pivots
At first, your toddler will explore moving their arm from their shoulder pivot. This will mean that their elbow will usually be straight and their wrist might look stiff, as the power of their movement is coming from the shoulder. These movements need lots of space. For example, if your child twirls a ribbon or makes a mark on paper, this will be with the whole arm moving from the shoulder. Over time you will notice that their shoulder will begin to provide stability and they will be able to pivot purposefully from their elbow. Elbow pivots still need lots of space – your toddler may enjoy sweeping the path, making large marks, pushing, pulling and climbing.

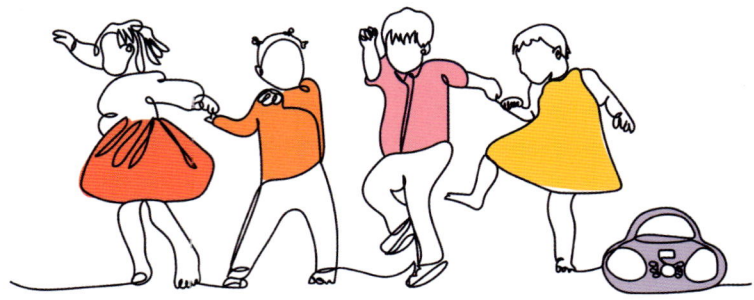

When your toddler pivots from their elbow you will notice that they still tend to keep their wrist quite stiff. The wrist pivot will take many years to fully master and your child will need lots of practice bending their wrists forwards, backwards and side to side, as well as rotating them.

Finding joy and expression in movement

Movement is also linked to emotions; in fact, the modern word 'emotion' stems from the Latin word emovere which means to move.

Rapid movements can increase your toddler's excitement and arousal, whilst slow movements have a calming effect. Our activities champion all the different ways in which big movements give your toddler the opportunity to express their emotions, perhaps through dance or alternatively through stamping and marching. We feel these fun and joyful moments are just as important as the whole-body learning they support.

> **It is recognised that physical play is a necessary part of development in all healthy mammals and that rough and tumble play seems to be a spontaneous urge stimulated from within the nervous system itself.**
>
> Sally Goddard Blythe[1]

QR code
Don't forget to scan this QR code to find lots more child development content and bonus activity ideas from the team at My First Five Years.

[1] Goddard Blythe, S. (2005), *The Well-Balanced Child: Movement and Early Learning*. Gloucestershire: Hawthorne Press.

Hide and seek
An obstacle treasure hunt

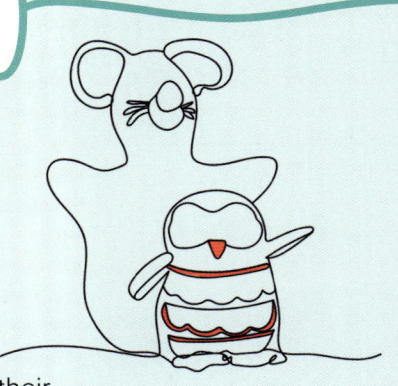

What you need:
- A selection of your toddler's favourite soft toys
- A basket or bag
- An outside space, such as a park or woodland

The steps:
- Encourage your toddler to choose a small collection of their favourite toys and explain that the toys are keen to play hide and seek!
- Head out to an outdoor space that provides lots of opportunities for hiding the toys on different levels, behind and under objects.
- Encourage your toddler to wait and close their eyes whilst you set up the hide and seek hunt.
- Hide toys on low-level surfaces, such as underneath a fallen tree trunk or behind a slide, to encourage your toddler to squat or kneel down to retrieve them.
- Hide some toys behind trees, bushes or walls to encourage your toddler to manoeuvre under, over or around an obstacle.
- Use higher surfaces to encourage your toddler to balance as they reach up. You could suspend a soft toy from a low branch or place it on top of a low wall.
- Explore with your toddler and encourage them to gather up their toys in a basket or bag.

Benefits for your toddler:
- Your toddler will be moving in lots of different ways to retrieve the toys, challenging their postural control and balance.
- As they reach and grasp, they will be strengthening the muscles of their upper body.

Building on:
- Include lots of positional language in the game, such as under, over, behind, up, down, next to and so on.

> ⚠ Ensure the space you play in is safe and secure for your toddler and do not allow them to explore unsupervised.

Twirling ribbon wands
Make some magic as you move

What you need:
- A stick
- A rubber band or elastic hair bobble
- Ribbons, old scarves or lengths of fabric
- Music (optional)

The steps:
- Ask your toddler to choose the ribbon they would like to attach to their wand.
- Tie or secure the ribbon to one end of the stick with the rubber band or hair bobble.
- If you can, make a second wand so you and your toddler have one each.
- Encourage your toddler to move in different ways by demonstrating different sorts of movements with the wand. Make waves, zig zags, circles, vertical up and down movements and horizontal movements which cross the mid-line of the body, twirls and leaps.
- Give your toddler the wand or if they already have one let them know they will be the leader in charge of the dance. Follow your child's lead and copy their movements with your own wand or hand.

Benefits for your toddler:
- The ribbon emphasises your movements and your toddler's movements, making them more visible.
- Helps your toddler to build strength, posture, balance and control as they move.
- Encourages your toddler to find the joy in moving spontaneously.

Building on:
- Make marks to represent the movements you have made by drawing them with a crayon on a large piece of paper.
- Take your ribbons outside on a windy day!
- Be as creative as you like as you develop your own dance routines – you may even find your toddler invents gestures to use in place of words, giving you a secret way to communicate through dance.

> Never leave your toddler unattended with long ribbons or string.

DIY window paint
Washable art

What you need:
- A low-level window or large plastic sheet, such as a shower curtain or plastic table covering
- A large mixing bowl and spoon
- Small containers for the paint
- A bucket of warm water and a cloth

For the paint:
- 1 cup (250ml) of plain flour
- 1 cup (250ml) of water
- ½ cup (125ml) of washing-up liquid
- Food colouring in whatever colour(s) you prefer

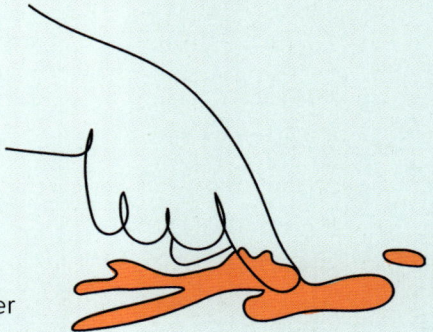

The steps:
- Encourage your toddler to help you to stir all of the ingredients for the paint together in the bowl, until the mixture is smooth and runny.
- Divide the mixture into the smaller containers and add one colour of food colouring to each container.
- If painting on a window, take the paint outside. You can also use the paint on a shower curtain on the floor or on a plastic table covering.
- Encourage your toddler to explore making marks on the window with whole-body movements, using their hands and fingers rather than a brush.
- Challenge them to reach high, cover the entire window or to copy some of your marks, such as zig zags, wavy lines and circles.
- Help your toddler to wash the paint away with the bucket of water and cloth so that they can paint again as many times as they like!

Benefits for your toddler:
- Stirring and mixing the ingredients employs larger muscles as your toddler pivots from the shoulder and elbow, along with smaller muscles in the hands and fingers.

Building on:
- Use the paints on tiled walls or a shower screen as an alternative to bath paints. Test on a small area first to ensure the natural dye does not stain your tiles or grout.

Swing ball challenge
Hit the ball as it moves

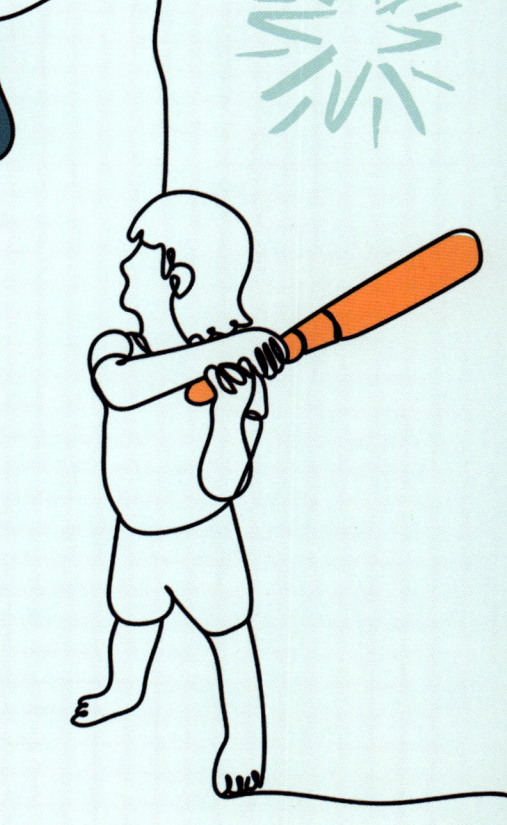

What you need:
- An old pair of tights
- Two small balls – tennis balls work well
- A washing line or low branch
- A child's bat or racquet

The steps:
- Cut the legs off the pair of tights.
- Drop one ball into each leg of the tights.
- Tie a knot in the ankle of the tights to hold the ball in place in the foot.
- Attach the tights to a washing line or the branch of a tree by tying or pegging them on; be sure to space them out so they don't get tangled together. Ensure the balls are at a low enough level to allow your toddler to succeed in hitting them.
- Encourage your toddler to take aim and hit the ball! Adjust the height as necessary.
- If you don't have space for this at home you could always take your swing ball with you to the park.

Benefits for your toddler:
- Watching the movement of the ball and taking aim is great for visual coordination.
- Supports your toddler's developing balance and upper-body coordination.

Building on:
- If you have more pairs of old tights, you could add swing balls of different lengths and with different sized balls.
- Adjust the size of the ball or the size of the bat – a larger bat and ball provides an easier challenge; a smaller bat and ball makes it more difficult.

Den making
Can you find your way in?

What you need:
- Large cardboard boxes, dining or garden chairs or a clothes airer
- Tarpaulin or large pieces of fabric, such as bed sheets or blankets
- A washing line
- Pegs or string
- Cushions and rugs

The steps:
- Begin by choosing a location for your den. This can be indoors or outdoors.
- Involve your toddler in this creative design process, let them lead the way.
- Test out different places, shapes and structures, such as under a table, between two chairs, or using a large box or a clothes airer as a support.
- Drape fabric or tarpaulin and peg or tie your various materials to provide a cover and shelter.
- Add some interior design details, such as cushions and rugs, to make a cosy space.
- Encourage your toddler to think about the route into their den. Can you both make a tricky or hidden route to the entrance? Perhaps a tunnel or something to crawl over or under and to keep the adults out!.

Benefits for your toddler:
- Develops upper body strength and dexterity as your toddler handles, organises and places the large props.
- Encourages a range of movements involving balance and coordination to build, enter and leave the den.

Building on:
- You could build a den outside with natural materials such as sticks, leaves, twigs and string.
- Your toddler can adapt and build on their perfect den design over time, adding or removing parts to make the den work for them. This builds their cognitive development through problem-solving and remembering information.

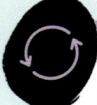

Use the den for different purposes throughout the day, such as settling down with a story before bedtime or using it for some role play in the morning.

Catch my tail
Running, chasing and dodging!

What you need:
- A long thin piece of fabric
- An open space, such as a garden, field or park

The steps:
- Tuck the long piece of fabric into your waistband so it hangs behind you like a tail.
- Challenge your toddler to grab your tail as you run. Encourage them to count one, two, three before setting off after you.
- Change direction or speed as your toddler gets close, but don't be too competitive! Let them catch you successfully after a few tries.
- When you have been caught you can swap over so that your toddler can tuck the fabric tail into their own waistband and you can chase them.

Benefits for your toddler:
- Builds fitness and muscle strength, balance and coordination as your toddler explores stopping, starting and changing direction.
- Large body movements help to develop your toddler's body awareness and spatial awareness (where their body is in space and in relation to other objects).

Building on:
- To increase the difficulty, make the tail a bit shorter by reducing the length of the fabric.
- Make the tail longer by having it touching the floor and challenge your toddler to place their foot on your tail to catch you, rather than grabbing it with their hand.

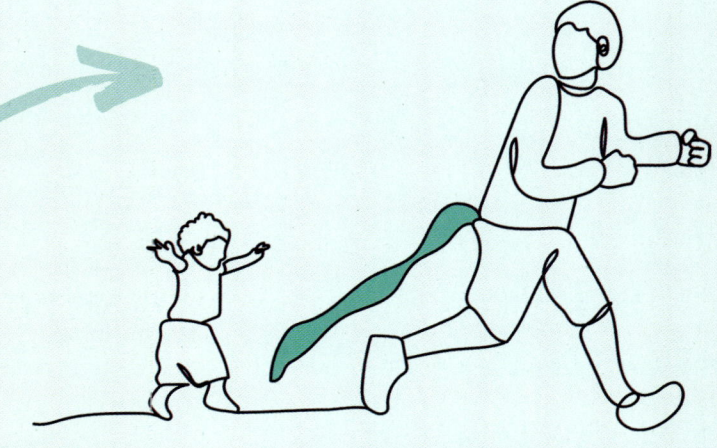

Washing day
Your own cleaning station

What you need:

- An outdoor space
- Wheeled or plastic toys, such as a balance bike, animals, dolls and bath toys
- A bucket
- Sponges, cloths and brushes
- Warm water
- Bubble bath
- Old towels
- Waterproofs and wellies (optional)

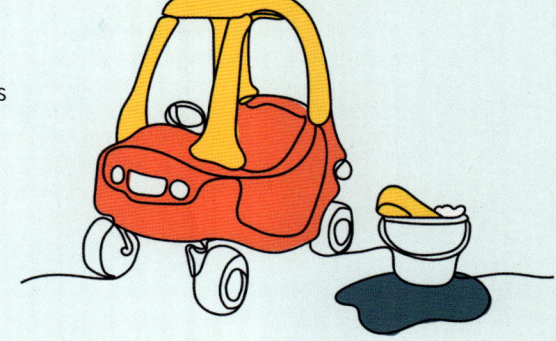

The steps:

- Help your toddler to organise a cleaning station outside. This could be an area marked out or simply a towel with the toys and bucket set out together.
- Support your toddler to mix the bubble bath with some warm water in the bucket and to carry it to the station.
- Use the sponges, cloths and brushes to wash the toys. Demonstrate how to wring excess water out of the cleaning tools.
- Describe your child's actions using positional and directional words, such as top, bottom, back, front, around, next to and so on.
- Dry the toys with the towel or leave them out in the sunshine to dry.

Benefits for your toddler:

- Balancing and using the two sides of the body together (bilateral coordination) can be developed when washing larger objects.
- Bending, reaching and stretching develops your toddler's strength, coordination and grasp.
- Arm, hand and finger strength and dexterity can be developed as your toddler wrings out the cloth, grips the sponge or turns on the tap.

Building on:

- Encourage your toddler to help you wash your car, bikes or other household items.

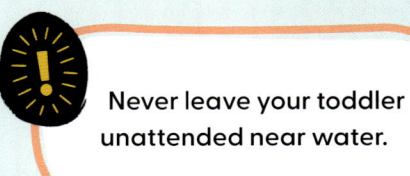

> Never leave your toddler unattended near water.

Peg up the clothes
Laundry time

What you need:
- Some damp laundry
- A laundry basket or bag
- A low-level washing line or clothes airer – this could be indoors or outdoors
- Pegs

The steps:
- Encourage your toddler to help you to pull the damp laundry out of the washing machine and put it in the laundry basket or bag.
- Damp laundry is heavy to carry and your toddler can help you to carry or pull the basket or bag ready to hang the clothing.
- Sort the clothing and demonstrate how to turn items that are inside out the right way round. Find matching socks!
- Your toddler can help you to peg up the washing on the low-level washing line or clothes airer, outside or inside.
- You can check together how the washing is drying. When it's dry, your toddler could help you to fold clothing and put it away in drawers or in wardrobes.

Benefits for your toddler:
- Your toddler is using their core muscles to support their posture as they work the muscles of their shoulders, arms, wrists and hands to pull the washing from the machine and carry or push it along in the basket or bag.
- Turning the washing the right way round and reaching to hang it involves your toddler developing and strengthening their larger muscles and their visual coordination when placing and pegging the items.

Building on:
- Helping with real-life chores can really motivate your child to get involved. Other activities that challenge the gross motor muscles are helping to make the bed, digging in the garden, cleaning the windows or vacuuming the house. It's a win-win situation for you both!

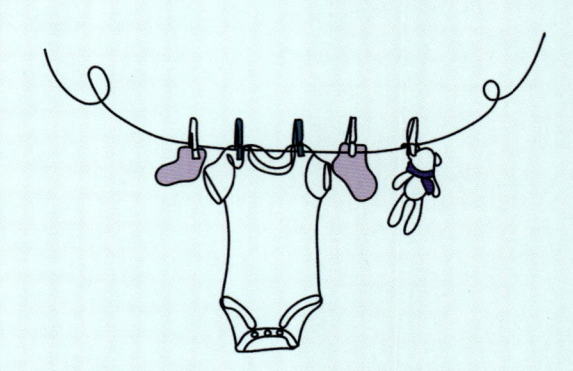

Ladder play
Step, jump and hop!

What you need:
- An outdoor space such as a woodland, field or park
- A collection of six to eight sturdy sticks about as long as your toddler's arm

The steps:
- Encourage your toddler to help you to collect the sticks.
- Together, lay the sticks down on the ground, equally placed as though they form the rungs of a ladder. Make the gap between each stick about twice as long as your toddler's foot.
- Challenge your toddler to step between the sticks as though climbing a ladder.
- After a few goes you can encourage your toddler to explore moving in different ways up and down the ladder. For example, jumping with two feet together, moving on all fours or side stepping. You could also add a time challenge for them to go up and back down as fast as they can.

Benefits for your toddler:
- Moving in different ways develops strength, coordination and balance.
- Encourages your toddler to develop spatial awareness and to consider and plan their movements to achieve the goal.

Building on:
- Make the ladder longer by adding more sticks or make the gaps between the sticks smaller.
- Make two ladders so your toddler can race you or a friend.
- Use larger sticks so that your toddler must jump over them.
- Make movement challenges more complex, such as hopping or travelling backwards.

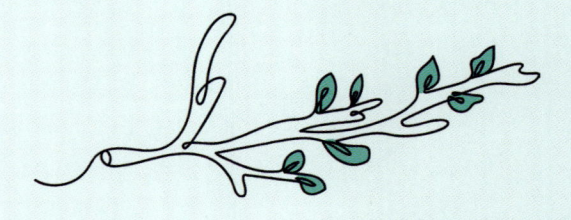

If your toddler enjoys this activity you can recreate it at home using masking tape or scarves, and make getting dressed into a game by having them put on an item of clothing when they jump to each new 'rung' of the ladder.

Who threw that?
Play catch like wild animals

What you need:

- An outdoor space
- A large, light ball, such as a well-inflated beach ball or plastic or foam football

The steps:

- Encourage your toddler to carry the ball outside to a safe area with space to throw.
- Let them practise throwing the ball freely to get used to how it moves and feels.
- Stand close by and ask your toddler to throw the ball to you so that you can try to catch it.
- Warn your toddler that you will throw it back and remind them how to hold their arms out ready.
- Throw the ball gently for your toddler to catch.
- Repeat a few times taking turns to throw and catch the ball.
- On one of your turns, tell your toddler that you're going to throw like a monkey. When you have told them this, throw the ball over-arm to your toddler.
- Encourage your toddler to copy your movement when they throw it back to you.
- Throw the ball to each other whilst pretending to be different animals, such as flapping the ball up and down like a bird before you throw, sliding it along the ground like a snake and throwing it from close to your chest like a gorilla. Let your toddler's imagination run free!
- Try to keep the focus on the funny ways of throwing rather than on how often the ball is caught.

Benefits for your toddler:

- Throwing in different ways will mean your toddler is adjusting the shape and force of their grip, helping them to build strength and confidence in grasping unusually shaped objects.

Building on:

- Take a step back after each throw to change the distance across which your toddler has to move the ball – they'll soon work out how to adjust their level of force to make the ball go further.

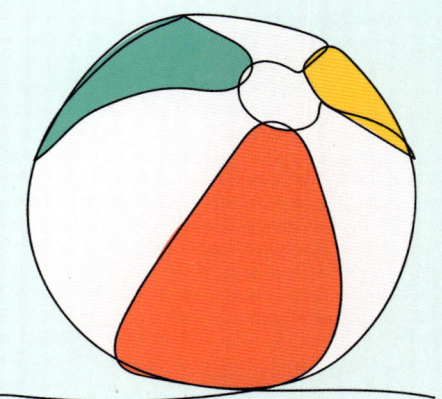

Chapter 3

Fine motor

Fine tuning movements

As your toddler learns to do more things for themselves, they will begin to coordinate both their fine and gross motor skills. Fine motor skills require the strength and coordination of the gross motor muscles in order to operate the smaller muscles in the body.

Fine motor skills are the ability to make small, detailed movements that involve using the tendons and cartilage in the wrists, hands, fingers and thumbs, along with many other small muscles including those found in the feet and in the face. These muscles all work together to build our fine motor skills.

Fine motor movements are often automatic and so slight that adults don't give much thought to them, however, they are complex and involve the coordination of the eyes, brain and muscles. Fine motor skills support the development of hand–eye coordination, object manipulation, dexterity and the overall coordination of your toddler's movements, which are all fundamental parts of physical development.

Building fine motor skills will give your toddler a growing sense of independence and satisfaction as they realise that they can complete daily activities themselves. For example, manipulating and handling their toys and equipment to achieve a goal when stacking bricks, controlling a ball, turning the pages of a book, making marks with a crayon or cutting with scissors.

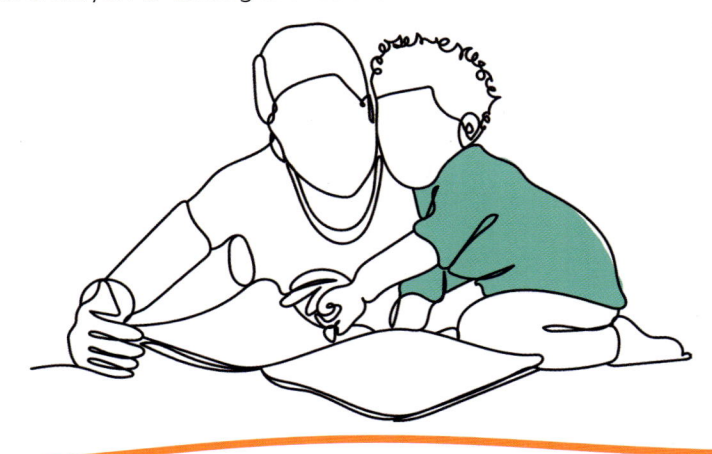

In addition, fine motor skills support your toddler to gain independence with daily care tasks, such as getting dressed, eating, brushing their hair or teeth, holding cutlery and drinking from a cup, all of which are very satisfying!

Your toddler will become more precise and successful in their movements over time as they practise these skills.

Developing palm arches

There are several arches in the palm of your toddler's hand which allow them to grip objects of different sizes and shapes. These affect the power of their grasp and also direct the movement of their fingers.

In-hand manipulation

In-hand manipulation is the skill of moving and positioning objects within one hand, without using the other hand to assist. Think about how your own hand can rotate marbles or how you can move an elastic band over different fingers. Your toddler will benefit from lots of practice manipulating objects of different shapes, sizes and weights.

Pincer grasp or grip

The pincer grasp or grip is the skill of being able to pick up small items using the end of the thumb and index finger, which allows the items to be manipulated effectively.

Bilateral coordination

Bilateral coordination is the ability to use both sides of the body at the same time. Many tasks that your toddler will want to do will require them to use this skill, and by developing bilateral hand coordination they will be able to complete fine motor tasks effectively. Sometmes this means both hands are doing the same thing, such as when your toddler claps or uses a rolling pin. Other actions will require them to alternate the movements of each side of the body in sequence, such as if they pull a rope, hand over hand. The most complex level of bilateral coordination is when each hand completes a different action, with one hand doing one job while the other hand does another. For example, when holding a piece of ribbon and cutting it with scissors or gripping a tube of tooth paste whilst rotating the lid.

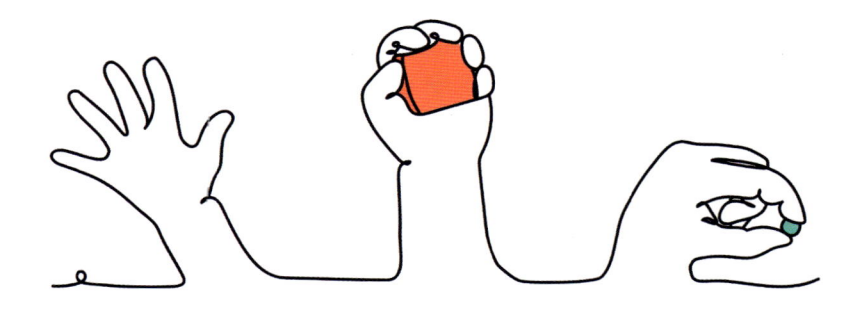

Finger isolation

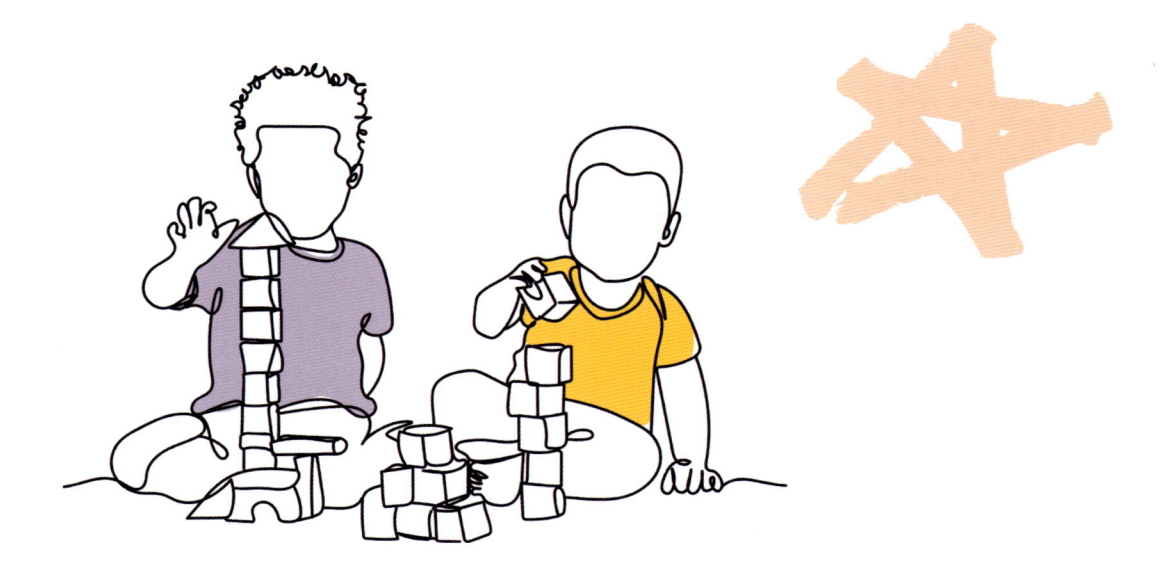

Finger isolation is the ability to use individual fingers, one at a time, to achieve a goal. This is an important skill because it allows your child to do many tricky tasks, such as closing zips, using scissors and holding a pencil.

Hand–eye coordination

Hand–eye coordination is also known as visual integration. Your toddler will be mastering the skill of controlling their hand movements guided by their vision, for example, to judge distance and speed to grasp a moving object, to thread a bead onto string, to pour water into a cup, to draw and to eat.

Hand dominance

Most people have a preference for using either their left or right hand. Your toddler will develop a dominant hand over time. Although they may seem to start to show a preference for a dominant hand, it is not possible to identify which hand it will be for certain until your child is older and they have more developed physical skills.

Oral motor skills

Developing the small muscles in your toddler's mouth supports their ability to control their breathing and carry out complex mouth movements, which in turn supports the development of language skills. These skills are challenged, for example, as they pucker their lips and blow bubbles and begin to babble and form their mouth into the different shapes needed to make words.

QR code

Don't forget to scan this QR code to find lots more child development content and bonus activity ideas from the team at My First Five Years.

Stone cairns
An ancient tradition to mark a special place

What you need:

- An outdoor space with readily available pebbles or stones
- A natural item to top your tower, such as a leaf, a shell or a conker

The steps:

- Explain to your toddler that you can mark a favourite place with a stone cairn. Choose a special spot to build.
- Spend some time collecting pebbles or small stones.
- Look carefully together at the shape and size of the pebbles or stones you have collected. Perhaps organise them by size.
- Encourage your toddler to think about which pebble or stone might be best on the bottom of a tower and discuss why this is, talking together about weight, size and shape.
- Support your child to manipulate and balance the stones as they build their tower upwards.
- Invite your toddler to place the special item right on the top of their cairn!

Benefits for your toddler:

- Your toddler will practise coordinating gross and fine motor skills as they gather and manipulate the stones, squat or bend to create a solid base, and move arms, hands and fingers to place the stones on the tower.
- Your toddler will develop thinking skills to plan movements to place and balance items on the tower that are not a regular shape.
- As your toddler grasps, manipulates and places each stone with precision and control, they are developing visual coordination.

Building on:

- Try stacking other natural items in different formations, such as creating a square shape with sticks by laying sticks parallel to each other on opposite sides of the square and building up.

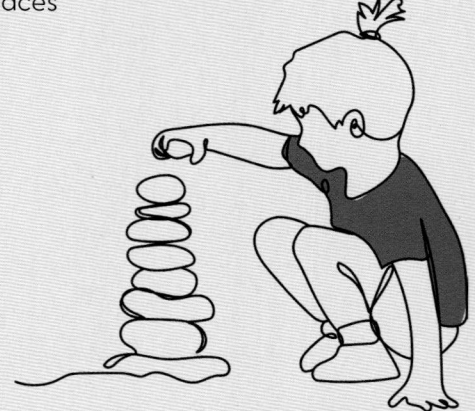

Threading tubes
Recycling hack!

What you need:
- Cardboard tubes from the middle of toilet or kitchen rolls
- Stiff string or ribbon

The steps:
- Cut up the cardboard tube to make rings of similar length pieces (start first with a tube with a wider diameter).
- Help your toddler to choose a comfortable position to start threading the cardboard rings onto the string or ribbon. They might prefer to stand, kneel or sit in order to rest their arms on a surface to provide stability as they thread.
- Help your toddler to tie one cardboard ring onto the end of the string or ribbon to stop the others from sliding off.
- Encourage them to hold the string or ribbon with one hand and to thread the rest of the cardboard rings on with the other hand. Demonstrate how to push the rings down to the end of the string.

Benefits for your toddler:
- Develops bilateral coordination as both hands are working together in coordination to achieve the task, although doing different jobs as one hand holds the tube and the other controls the string.
- Strengthens finger muscles and pincer grip.
- Develops visual perception as your toddler coordinates information from their eyes with movement of their hands.

Building on:
- Your toddler could decorate the cardboard rings by painting or drawing on them. These could then be used to decorate a den or could be attached to a pull-along toy.

> Stay close to your toddler when they are using ribbon or string, and never let them wrap it around their neck or head.

Cutting tray
Snip it up!

What you need:

- A tray and a selection of plastic containers or a cutlery draw tray with multiple sections
- Child-sized scissors
- Items to cut up, such as lengths of ribbon, strips of paper, strips of card, toilet roll tubes, paper straws and natural items, such as grass or leaves

The steps:

- Set up the tray with the scissors in one section and the different materials to snip in the other sections or containers.
- Encourage your child to explore cutting the materials. If necessary, demonstrate how to open and close the scissors and then open them again ready for the next snip.
- Your toddler might need your support at first to help them to hold the paper or material to be snipped steady, whilst they focus on the scissor skill. Gradually they will be able to use both hands in coordination.

Benefits for your toddler:

- Develops wrist, hand and finger strength when opening and closing the scissors.
- Develops bilateral coordination – cutting involves each hand doing different tasks. The preferred hand uses the scissors and the other hand turns the paper or material.

Building on:

- As your toddler masters the skill of cutting with one snip, you could offer wider pieces of paper or card to encourage the need for more snips to reach the other side and cut through.

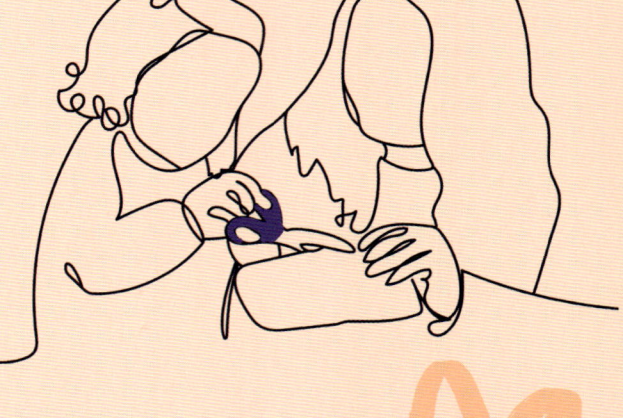

Never leave your toddler unsupervised with scissors.

Sand stories
Drawing in the ground

What you need:

- A large tray, such as a garden tray, baking tray or serving tray – preferably a plain colour or you could place some coloured paper on the tray
- Dry sand or any other sensory material, such as powder paint, dry soil or any out-of-date flour, salt, spices or lentils
- Fingers! Plus tools, such as a pastry brush, paint brush, shaving brush, sticks of different sizes, a fork or a comb
- Other natural items your child might want to add to their sand picture, such as leaves, stones or twigs

The steps:

- Tip a small layer of sand or your chosen sensory material onto the tray and spread out evenly.
- Demonstrate to your toddler how to use their index finger to make marks and tracks in the sand. Your child may prefer to use all of their fingers or their whole hand to explore. Comment on the types of lines or shapes you and they make.
- Encourage your toddler to tell their own story in the sand; they might create a wavy line to represent the sea or a circle for a face, and so on.
- You could encourage your toddler to also use the tools to explore different sorts of marks in the sand and they could incorporate the natural items to add to their story.

Benefits for your toddler:

- Encourages finger isolation skills as the index finger is used.
- Develops awareness of how gross and finer movements link to the corresponding marks by making your toddler's movements visible in the sand. Some larger movements might come from the shoulder or elbow, smaller movements from the wrist, hand and fingers.
- Supports hand–eye coordination.
- Develops the ability to grasp and control tools and the ability to manipulate smaller items as your toddler picks up and places items in the sand.

Building on:

- With careful supervision, old framed mirrors or picture frames make a satisfying tray.
- Notice where your toddler is pivoting from in their movements. Are they working from the shoulder, elbow, wrist or fingers? If they are enjoying large movements, ensure the tray is large enough to accommodate these.

Whittling away
Safe knife skills

What you need:

- A vegetable peeler
- A root vegetable, such as a carrot or a potato, or a dry bar of soap (optional)
- A twig or branch that is soft and easy to carve, such as silver birch, willow, sycamore, alder or lime
- A child-sized chair
- Sandpaper for smoothing rough edges (optional)

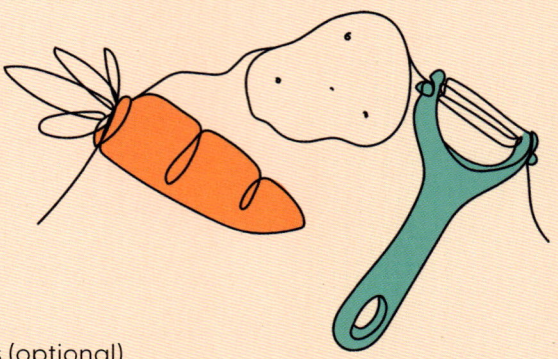

The steps:

- Your toddler may find it helpful to practise using the peeler on vegetables or a dry bar of soap before they get started on the wood.
- Help your toddler to sit on the chair with both legs to one side and the branch held to the other side, angled down towards the floor. So, if they prefer to use their right hand, they should sit with their legs to the left-hand side and the branch past their knees to the right-hand side. For safety reasons, their hands should not be between their legs or in their lap.
- Demonstrate how to hold the branch steady with the supporting hand, and how to use a pushing downwards stroke with the other hand to peel away from the body and the hand holding the wood.
- Encourage your toddler to be patient and to aim for a little bit of bark to be removed at a time. Enjoy discovering together what lies beneath.
- If using sandpaper, support your toddler to sand any rough edges.

Benefits for your toddler:

- Your toddler will be developing bilateral coordination as they use one hand to peel and the other to grasp the wood to hold it steady.

Building on:

- Your toddler can help you peel the vegetables for mealtimes.

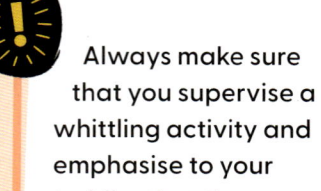

> Always make sure that you supervise a whittling activity and emphasise to your toddler that they must be seated when using the peeler.

Taste-safe paint
Squeezy bottle painting

What you need:
- A mixing bowl and large spoon
- Empty squeezy bottles, such as washing up liquid bottles or ketchup bottles
- Small bowls or plastic containers and a teaspoon
- A large sheet of paper (perhaps an old roll of wall paper) or a wide tray
- For the paint:
  - 250ml of corn flour
  - 250ml of cold water
  - 750ml of hot water
  - Food colouring – natural varieties are available

The steps:
- Encourage your toddler to help you to mix the cornflour with cold water in the mixing bowl to form a paste.
- Carefully add the hot water to the paste and stir.
- Divide up the mixture into the small bowls or plastic containers and add drops of a different food colour to each portion. Encourage your toddler to help choose the colours and to stir the food colouring into each mixture using the teaspoon.
- Allow your mixtures to cool and then spoon them into the empty squeezy bottles.
- Encourage your toddler to use both hands to squeeze the bottles. Adjust the consistency of the paint by adding more water if your toddler finds it difficult to squeeze hard enough for the mixture to flow out.
- Let your toddler get creative, squeezing the paint onto the paper or into the tray.

Benefits for your toddler:
- Mixing the paint encourages bilateral coordination as your toddler holds the bowl with one hand whilst mixing with the other.
- Using both hands to squeeze the mixture out of the bottle develops strength in the palm arches and fingers, whilst also using larger muscles of the arm and shoulder to guide the paint around the paper or tray.

Building on:
- Try the same activity outside with a squeezy bottle filled with water.

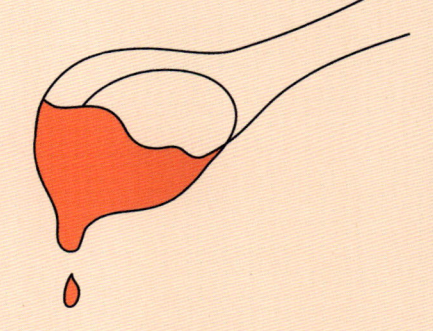

> Always make sure your toddler is safe when you are using or pouring hot water.

Dough play
Workout for the wrists, hands and fingers

What you need:
- A football-sized portion of play dough – we are going big!
- For the play dough:
    * Two cups (500ml) plain flour
    * ½ cup (125ml) salt
    * 2 cups (500ml) hot water
    * 2 tbsp oil
    * 2 tbsp cream of tartar
- A mixing bowl and a large spoon
- A surface to play on, such as a low table, a large tray or a chopping board

The steps:
- Encourage your toddler to help you to mix together the flour, salt, cream of tartar and oil in a large bowl.
- Slowly add the hot water to the dry mixture until it has just combined.
- When the mixture has cooled sufficiently, your toddler can help you to stir continuously until it becomes sticky and doughy.
- Encourage your toddler to take the mixture out of the bowl and place it on the surface. Help them to knead the dough until it binds together.
- The dough is ready to play with! Your toddler can explore kneading, squeezing, pushing, pulling, twisting, patting and poking the dough. Demonstrate different ways of manipulating the dough, such as rolling a sausage or making a ball.

Benefits for your toddler:
- Encourages bilateral movements when carrying out actions such as mixing whilst holding the bowl, twisting and pulling the dough, rolling the dough into a ball or sausage and pushing down on the dough with both hands.
- Develops grasp and pincer grip when your toddler is picking up large and small pieces of dough.

Building on:
- Enhance play by incorporating some tools, such as rolling pins and cutters.

> ⚠ Always make sure your toddler is safe when you are using or pouring hot water.

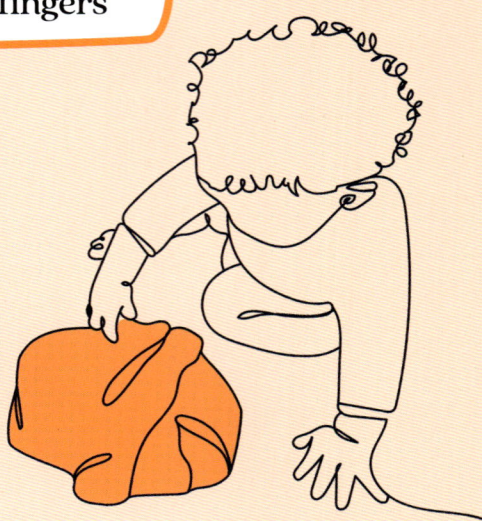

Match of the day
Blow football

What you need:
- Tissue paper or newspaper
- PVA glue or a glue stick
- Paint brush (optional)
- A table or space on the floor
- Cushions or books (optional)
- Two cardboard tubes
- Two old birthday or Christmas cards
- Scissors

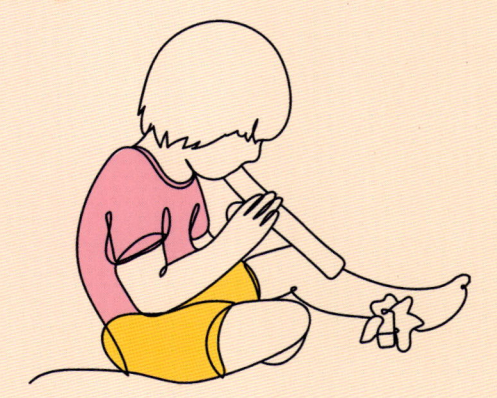

The steps:
- Encourage your toddler to help you to rip the tissue paper or newspaper into small pieces.
- Put a little glue on the paper and crumple and squeeze it together to make a small ball, a little smaller than a golf ball. If you are using PVA glue you could brush some on the outside of the ball.
- Whilst the glue is drying, set up your football pitch by creating a space on the table or floor. You could create barriers around the edge of the space with cushions or books.
- Take a cardboard tube each and challenge your toddler to blow through the tube to move the ball to the end of the pitch whilst you attempt to blow it back the other way!
- Add to the challenge by making a goal at each end by lying the old birthday card on its long edges and cutting out a rectangle shape from the front.

Benefits for your toddler:
- Supports bilateral coordination as your toddler rips the paper and manipulates it to form the ball.
- Develops oral motor skills – puckering the lips and blowing works the small muscles in your toddler's mouth.

Building on:
- Reduce the scale and increase the challenge by using paper straws and smaller rolled-up balls of paper.
- You could add a whistle for more blowing practice and to ensure there is no foul play!

Scoop and splash
Filling, pouring and transferring water

What you need:

- A large shallow tray or container, such as a baking tray or a plastic tub
- A large towel
- Water and a few drops of food colouring – natural varieties are available
- A variety of smaller empty containers with handles, such as jugs, plastic cups, milk cartons and plastic bottles
- Spoons of different sizes, ladles or measuring spoons

The steps:

- Place the shallow tray or container on the floor, indoors or outdoors, somewhere where your toddler has space to play. Place a towel under the tray to catch splashes.
- Put some water in the tray and add a few drops of food colouring.
- Set up the range of containers and place the spoons and ladles alongside.
- Encourage your toddler to explore the water using the containers, spoons and ladles.
- Watch how they play. They may scoop up the water and tip the containers to watch the flow start and stop, transfer the water from one container to another, experiment with splashing and lots more!

Benefits for your toddler:

- Your toddler will use different hand movements to grip and scoop, and the different handles will provide a workout for the muscles in their wrists, hands and fingers.
- They will use visual coordination to move water between containers and to scoop using the spoons.

Building on:

- Use smaller containers and spoons for a harder challenge, or larger containers and spoons for an easier challenge.
- Cut off the neck of a plastic bottle to make a funnel to use when pouring the water into the containers.

Never leave your toddler unattended near water.

Hammering
Real-life skills

What you need:

- A hammer suitable for a toddler – small, light hammers are available which are easier to use and safer for toddlers
- Something to hammer, such as:
  * Nails – round 25mm nails with a smooth shaft and large head are ideal
  * Golf tees
- Something to hammer into, such as:
  * A soft patch of ground outside
  * Soft wood, such as balsa wood blocks

The steps:

- Demonstrate to your toddler how to hold the hammer – by the centre of the handle, in their preferred hand.
- Show them how to hold the nail or golf tee with the finger and thumb of their supporting hand and how to place it on the ground or wood, ready to be hammered. You might need to hold the nail or item for them.
- Encourage your toddler to test out gentle taps with the hammer at first as they become accustomed to the movement and force required. Remind them to always look at what they are doing.
- After a few knocks, see if the nail or golf tee can stand up on its own when you move your hand away.

Benefits for your toddler:

- They will use visual coordination and spatial awareness to adjust movements to hit the target with accuracy.
- Hammering involves gross and fine motor skills.

Building on:

- You could find items with holes in, such as large buttons, or make holes in plastic lids for your child to attach to the wood using the nails.

> ⚠ Always supervise your toddler when they are using tools and explain to them that they are only safe to use when with you or another adult. Count out how many nails you have, and count again at the end, to make sure they are all safely packed away.

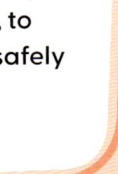

Chapter 4

Sensory

Making sense of it all

Your toddler's senses began to develop in the womb, and since birth the senses have continued to develop as your toddler explores the world and encounters new experiences. Each of your toddler's senses are linked to receptors in different parts of their body which send signals to their brain.

Sensory development is not only about the development of these receptors, but also about the development of the areas of the brain that process this information. Over time, and with plenty of practice, your toddler's brain will begin to filter and sift through the overwhelming number of messages that arrive, learning to discard those that are not relevant and to focus on those that really matter.

Your toddler's filter is still fairly wide open as they have not had enough experience to discern the things that really matter, as such, they may appear distractible. This is because they are often pulled to switch their attention between all sorts of things, especially things that are novel or very appealing. Your filter by contrast will be more fixed, so when going for a walk, for example, you are less likely to stop and examine the detail of everything.

The development of your toddler's senses is key as they begin to work together to underpin other areas of development, such as supporting the gross and fine motor skills. For example, being able to balance when moving and lifting items, building cognitive understanding of their body and the space it's in and developing an understanding of the social skills (and rules) they're learning.

As your toddler is now mobile, they will be embarking on a period of busy exploration and discovering new sensations. Their sensory receptors, including their eyes, nose and skin, then send messages to their brain to help them to make sense of what they are experiencing. This will also help to keep them safe, which is especially important at this stage of busy activity! For example, they will react when they feel the cold water of a puddle or hear the sound of a vehicle approaching.

Many people are aware of the five key external senses: touch, hearing, smell, taste and sight. But there are many other senses, including three lesser-known internal senses, which are at play for your toddler. These are the proprioceptive sense, the vestibular sense and interoceptive awareness.

Your toddler will be supported to develop their five **external** senses:

Touch

Touch plays a big role in the sensory information your toddler receives and the skin is the largest sense organ. Touch can help us to understand pressure, texture, pain, hot and cold. Touch is important when bonding with your toddler, and much of the day-to-day care you give your toddler provides an opportunity to positively support their emotions through touch. For example, when you soothe them through cuddles, hold their hand to provide reassurance or pat them to calm them for sleep. However, touch is complex and it is interesting to note that people vary in their capacity to tolerate touch and may, for example, be sensitive to being touched or to being touched on particular parts of the body.

Touch also plays a big role in your toddler's exploration as they discover the world by actively touching the things around them. The most sensitive areas for the reception of touch are their hands, fingers, mouth and tongue.

Hearing

Hearing will allow your toddler to notice a sound, to try to gauge whether it is important amongst background noise, to locate where it is coming from and perhaps to decide whether or not they have heard it before. They may even set off to try and find the source of the sound!

Familiar sounds such as birdsong, the doorbell and your voice will now be identified easily, but unfamiliar sounds may startle or surprise your toddler. Hearing keeps your toddler safe as they listen out for cars when crossing the road or hear your voice and respond when you call them to stop.

Your toddler will also be developing their range of speech sounds as they listen to the sounds of their native language and begin to try to replicate these by producing their own sounds. They will rely on plenty of auditory feedback as they test new words and match their sounds to the sounds you and others make.

Smell

The receptors for smell react to the odours around us. Scientists believe that these are found not only in the nose but also beyond, such as in the respiratory tract and the gut. Smell receptors help to tell your toddler what is good and safe to eat and also to alert to other dangers. Bad smells or smells associated with something negative can provide warning – for example, the smell of food that is no longer fresh provides a warning not to eat it and the smell of smoke alerts us to the possibility of fire.

Smell is strongly associated with taste, so plays a big part in your toddler's developing tastes for different foods and drinks. Smell also has an emotional element as it can be associated with triggering strong memories.

Taste

The sense of taste works in combination with the sense of smell. There are an important set of receptors on your toddler's tongue – little bumps with millions of cells – known as taste buds. These receptors trigger neural signals in the brain and start the digestive process. Your toddler's sense of taste, combined with other senses, will tell them about flavours, texture and temperature, and will help them to decide their food preferences.

Your toddler will be developing their sense of taste every day through experiencing different foods, and their taste buds play a key role in making sure they get the nutrition they need. Children are big fans of sweet foods as they recognise sugar as being a high-energy food which their bodies seek out in order to grow. They might also become a little more selective when eating now that they're on the move. Toddlers are very sensitive to bitter tastes because in nature bitterness might indicate a poisonous food, and now that your toddler can move freely, their sense of taste is trying to protect them from eating any potentially harmful foods (or plants) they find on their travels.

Sight

Your toddler's sense of sight, along with their other senses, is helping them to form their own view of the world. As they look at the things around them, their brain will be combining information about shape, colour, size, depth, movement and distance.

Your toddler will be linking what they see to their movements as they work out how it looks and feels when they move their body, and how their body moves in relation to the space around it – this links to their internal sense of proprioception. This is a life skill which comes with the development of depth perception – the ability to understand the size and depth of what you see, and spatial awareness – the ability of your brain to take that information about size and depth and understand how it relates to you or the objects around you that need to move into the space.

Your toddler's eyesight is now well developed, meaning they can see into the distance and in detail, however, the way they process what they see is still developing and will continue to do so as they grow. Skills such as being able to reliably pick out and recognise small details in busy scenes (known as visual discrimination) are only believed to reach adult levels after several years, with some research suggesting around school age and other research suggesting even later, so you will need to help your toddler to make sense of these details in the meantime.

Using vision to make sense of 'non-verbal' cues, such as pointing or moving your own gaze to something, helps your toddler to channel their attention as they bring their gaze to things of interest, for example, whilst looking at details in a picture book and as they 'shift their gaze', for example, when looking at something far away in the distance.

Your toddler will be supported to develop their **internal** senses:

The proprioceptive sense

The proprioceptive sense, sometimes referred to as body awareness, tells your toddler where their body parts are in relation to other body parts and how their body's position relates to the space around it. The proprioceptive sense is linked to receptors in your toddler's muscles and joints; these receptors are stimulated by movement and pressure, so pulling, jumping, swinging and hugging all provide proprioceptive input. Experiencing lots of proprioceptive input allows your toddler to develop a detailed internal body map so they can understand their relative size and position in the world and how to interact with the space around them, which will continue to change and adapt as they grow.

As adults we can usually make familiar movements without looking at them, or thinking much about them, such as when you reach for and pick up a mug while looking at something else (perhaps this book!). But toddlers are still in the process of learning about depth, distance, where their body starts and ends and how to judge the space between objects, so they need lots of practice and sensory input to get to grips with this.

The proprioceptive sense is important, and working hard, particularly during the toddler years as your child seeks information to maintain balance and posture as they 'find their feet' and begin to walk upright or run on two legs.

The vestibular sense

The vestibular sense is sometimes known as our balance centre. It is primarily located in our inner ear. The brain receives information about body movements from receptors in our inner ear, then works with our other senses to help us to stay balanced. Your toddler will have developed this sense as a baby when they were rocked, bounced, picked up and carried. Now, as your toddler prepares to make a movement, they will rely on sensory information to anticipate what their body needs to do, and the vestibular sense enables them to coordinate their movements, for example, to move up or down a step, to navigate around an obstacle or to throw a ball at a target. This sense is fine-tuned through trial and error so that your toddler's brain can develop patterns that allow them to smoothly carry out actions.

> **Soon after taking their first steps, you may notice your toddler often seems determined to unsteady themselves again as they seek out opportunities to make themselves dizzy by spinning, swinging or tipping themselves upside down. They naturally seek these sensations that help organise the brain.**
>
> Alistair Bryce-Clegg

Interoceptive awareness

Interoceptive awareness helps your toddler to understand what is happening inside their body, for example, when they feel hot or cold, hunger, pain, the need to go to the toilet and feelings associated with emotions. Your toddler will continue to develop an awareness of these sensations right into adulthood.

During the toddler years, the sense of interoception helps your child to begin to manage their own health and care needs. For example, they may be able to anticipate when they need to use the toilet though familiarity with the sensations they experience in their body, which might manifest themselves as changes in concentration or being unable to sit still. Similarly, they will grow to understand when they are feeling hungry or when they are full, or even when they are tired!

The activities in this book will help your toddler to explore, test and understand the sensory feedback that they receive from different experiences in safe and playful ways.

QR code

Don't forget to scan this QR code to find lots more child development content and bonus activity ideas from the team at My First Five Years.

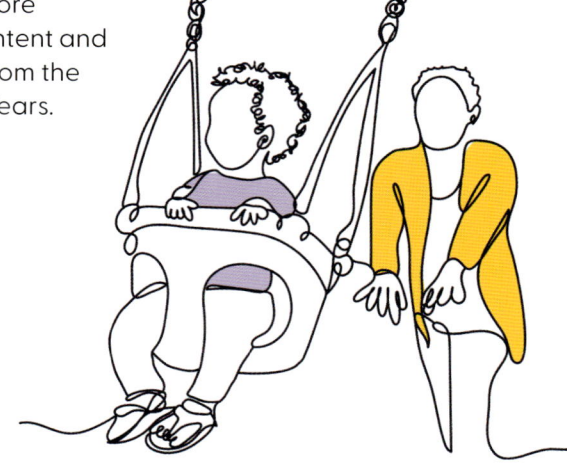

Make some whizzy noise
A cardboard tube kazoo

What you need:
- A cardboard tube from a kitchen roll
- A pencil
- Decorating materials, such as crayons, felt-tip pens or paint
- Baking or greaseproof paper
- Scissors
- Elastic bands to fit tightly around the tube

The steps:
- Holding your cardboard tube steady on its side, make three holes adjacent to each other towards one end of the tube. To do this, poke the tip of the pencil through the cardboard tube – turn the pencil round a few times to widen the hole. Leave around two fingers width between the end of the tube and the holes.
- Encourage your toddler to decorate the tube using crayons, felt-tip pens or paint.
- Cut a square of the baking paper and secure it over the end of the tube closest to the holes using the elastic bands. Don't cover the holes with the paper or band.
- Encourage your toddler to have a go at playing their kazoo. They will need to put their mouth against the open end of the tube to create a seal and then make a sound. This might take a bit of practice and it may be helpful to demonstrate first. Don't worry about what sounds they are making – the more creative their noises are the better!
- When you are making sounds with the kazoo, your toddler could hold the other end of tube close to their ear or touch the paper gently, to allow them to feel the vibrations as well as hearing the sounds.
- Encourage your toddler to try out different noises; repeating sounds such as 'doo, doo' or 'laa, laa' works well.

Benefits for your toddler:
- Your toddler will explore how moving their mouth in different ways changes the type and volume of the sound they produce.
- Your toddler will be using their sense of hearing and touch as they feel vibrations in the tube linked to the sounds that are produced.

Building on:
- Try tubes of different lengths and widths to test out the sorts of noise that can be made.

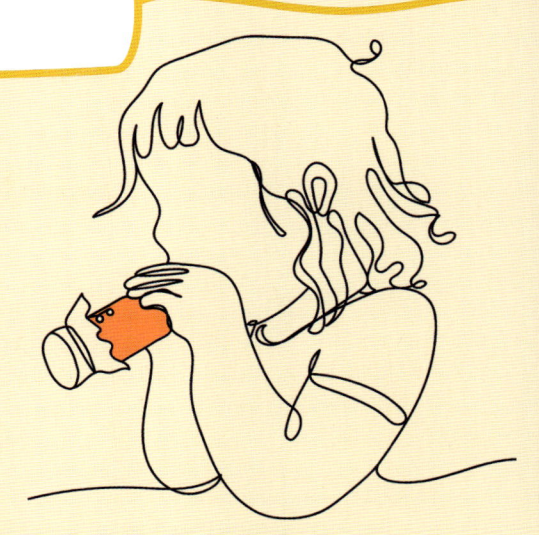

Musical statues and bumps
Freeze when the music stops!

What you need:

- A music player with some favourite songs
- Some space in your home for moving around or dancing

The steps:

- Explain the simple rules of the game musical statues to your toddler. When the music is playing, they can move around or dance. When the music stops, they must 'freeze' and stand as still as a statue.
- Have a few practice turns by beginning to play the music and then pausing it suddenly. Vary the length of time you play the music before stopping it.
- You could playfully check if your toddler is completely still by walking around them or trying to make them laugh!
- Repeat this a few times.
- Change the rules a little by explaining that it's now musical bumps and your toddler must sit down quickly on the floor when the music stops.
- You could encourage your toddler to place their hand on their chest to feel how their heart rate rises after exercise and point out how their breathing also changes.

Benefits for your toddler:

- Your toddler is developing the ability to tune in to the music, listening and remaining alert to the sounds as they move.
- Standing still develops your toddler's vestibular and proprioceptive sense, especially if they are caught in an unusual position as the music stops!
- Your toddler's understanding of their internal sensations will grow as they feel the changes in their body.

Building on:

- Try playing the game with a group.
- You could add to the challenge by taking turns to make up your own rules about what happens when the music stops – for example, putting your hand on your head or balancing on one leg!

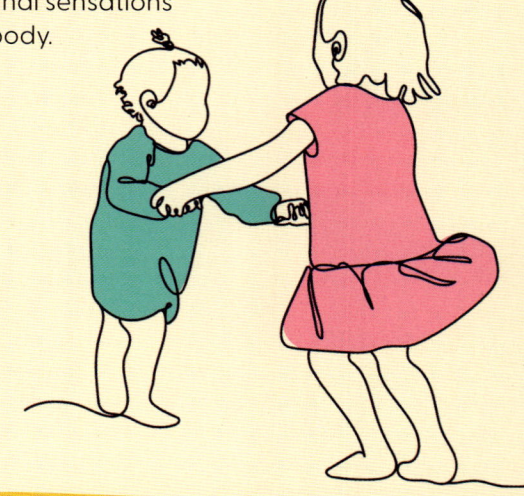

Roll me, watch me, stop me
Catch the chaos

What you need:
- Toys or objects that will roll, such as wheeled toys, balls or empty cylindrical bottles
- A large empty box

The steps:
- Lie the box on its side with the opening towards you and your toddler.
- Tell your toddler that they can stand or sit wherever they like when you start to roll a toy. This might be next to you, in front of you or in front of the box.
- Let your toddler know they will be trying to stop the rolling objects from getting into the box.
- Move a little way away from your toddler and start rolling your items, one at a time.
- Start by rolling them gently to give your toddler a good chance to grab the toys. If they find it tricky, encourage them to try standing or sitting in a different spot, closer to the box.
- Swap roles so that your toddler has the opportunity to try rolling the toys into the box.
- Play this game as many times as your toddler wants to – the more they play the better they will become at predicting how to move in order to catch the object.

Benefits for your toddler:
- Watching and catching moving objects helps your toddler to synchronise body movements with their vision – this will help to integrate their senses and develop hand–eye coordination.
- Rolling items helps to develop the gross motor skills needed for pivoting from the arm and shoulder, and the fine motor skills needed for moving and gripping objects. These are both important abilities for life skills such as writing and getting dressed.

Building on:
- You can use a larger box so that your toddler has to think about covering more of the area when catching the item.
- You can start by using fairly large items that are easy to grab, and then move towards smaller and smaller items as your toddler gets to grips with the game. Small items will challenge their hand–eye coordination more than large ones.
- You can play outside where a sloped surface, or the wind, can change the direction of the object, adding another challenge for your toddler's senses.

Whisk it up
Bubble beards and wigs

What you need:

- A bath, a large bowl, a bucket or a shallow tray
- Water
- Bubble bath
- A home-made play kit of tools for mixing, stirring and whisking, such as a balloon whisk, a range of metal, wood or plastic spoons or a handheld rotary whisk
- Paper straws

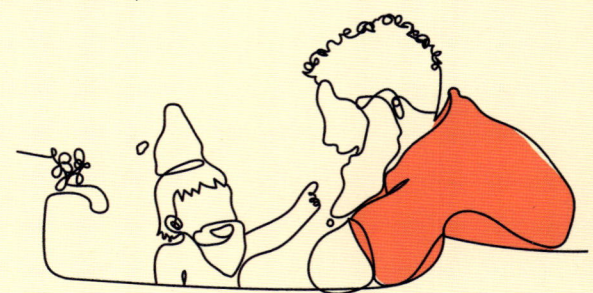

The steps:

- Encourage your toddler to help you to run the bath or to fill your container with water. Add the bubble bath.
- Join in playing with your toddler testing out the different utensils in your play kit. Demonstrate how to move the water around and whisk up some more bubbles.
- Use the paper straws by placing one end under the water and blowing through the other end to make some more bubbles rise up. It can take time for toddlers to learn how to blow, instead of sucking, through a straw. If your toddler is likely to try and drink the water instead of blowing bubbles, use the straw yourself instead of letting them have a turn.
- When you have plenty of bubbles you could scoop some up to make yourself and your toddler a bubble beard or even a bubble wig!

Benefits for your toddler:

- Your toddler will be exploring the water and the bubbles by touch, sight and smell.

Building on:

- You can add to the bath play kit with other household items, such as sieves, strainers, colanders, spoons with holes in, plastic funnels, bowls and bottles.

> ⚠️ Never leave your toddler unattended near water and always check the water temperature is safe before your toddler has access to it.

Squeezy sensory dough
Play dough with a twist

What you need:
- For your play dough:
  - 500ml (2 cups) baking powder
  - 375ml (1½ cups) warm water
  - 250ml (1 cup) cornflour
- A mixing bowl and spoon
- A pan and heat source
- A plate or baking paper
- Fresh lavender or a bunch of fresh herbs, such as mint, thyme or sage (optional)

The steps:
- Encourage your toddler to mix the dry ingredients together in a mixing bowl and then to gradually add the warm water. Transfer your mixture to the pan.
- Place your pan over a medium heat and warm gently, stirring continuously until the mixture thickens.
- Spoon the dough out onto the baking paper or a plate and use the spoon to fold and press the dough. Do not touch it with your hands as it will be hot.
- Allow to cool and then knead the dough a little more to ensure it is smooth.
- Now your toddler can explore the texture of the play dough. Using cornflour gives the dough a smoother more rubbery texture than standard play dough.
- Give your toddler lots of time to explore squeezing, squashing and shaping the dough with their hands.
- If you choose to, offer the selection of herbs or lavender to your toddler to add to their play dough.

Benefits for your toddler:
- Playing with play dough provides a great tactile activity and the addition of herbs and lavender enhances the sensory experience.

Building on:
- When you are out and about you could forage for other natural items to add to your play dough, such as flower petals, leaves or bark.

> Always supervise your toddler around a heat source and do not allow them to touch the play dough until it has cooled to a touch-safe temperature.

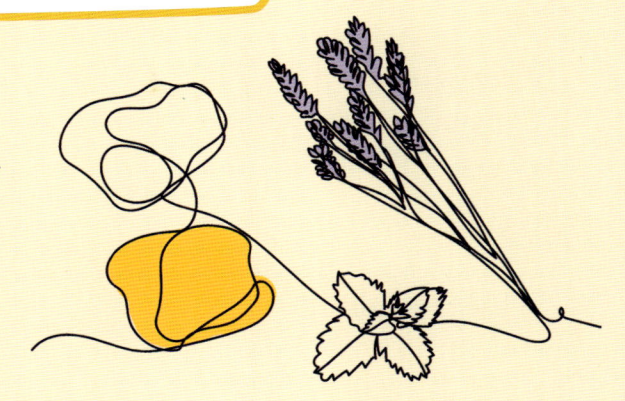

Whose voice is that?
Storytime with family and friends

What you need:

- A smart phone
- A friend or family member

The steps:

- Ask your friend or family member to say a short 'guess who' message for your toddler (without revealing who they are) whilst you record their voice on your smart phone. Or they can send the message via a messaging service.
- Play the voice recording to your toddler and see if they can recognise who is talking.
- You could then record your toddler's voice so that they can send a message back.

Benefits for your toddler:

- This activity will help your toddler to tune into and recognise familiar voices.
- It will also give them the opportunity to hear their own voice recorded.

Building on:

- You can adapt this activity and personalise the messages, perhaps encouraging grandparents to record themselves reading a bedtime story or singing a rhyme.
- When your toddler gets good at recognising familiar voices, you could ask the person leaving the voice note to do so in a silly voice – perhaps pretending to be a bear with a growling voice or a tiny mouse with a high pitched voice. Challenge your toddler to guess whose voice it is.

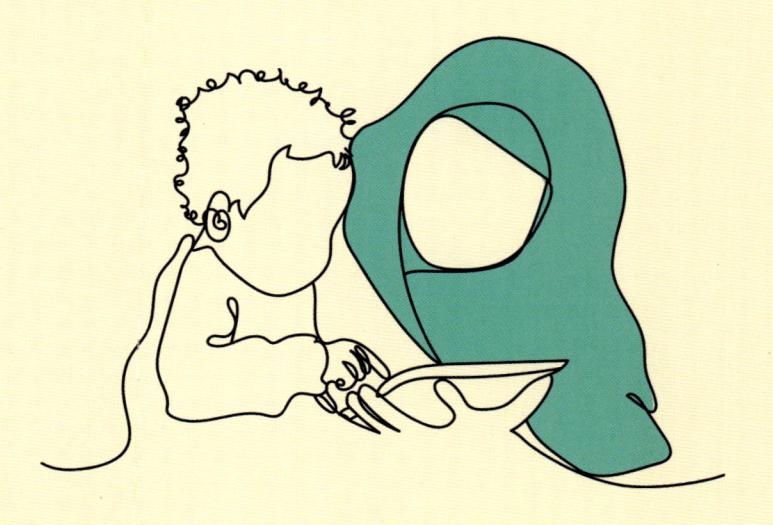

Light and dark
Playing with shadows

What you need:

- A light source – outside this could be the sun, inside a torch or lamp
- A screen – outside this could be a bedsheet suspended from a washing line or a stretch of pavement or wall where you can see your shadow, inside a curtain pulled flat or an empty expanse of wall
- Natural items, such as a feather, a long blade of grass or a flower
- A selection of small toys, such as toy animals, diggers, trains and wooden blocks

The steps:

- Position yourself and your toddler between the home-made screen (or wall/pavement) and the light source so that you create shadows with your bodies.
- Encourage your toddler to experiment with the different shapes and shadows they can make as they move their body in different ways, such as lifting their arms up overhead or out to the sides, standing on one leg and so on.
- You can also experiment with smaller movements using hands and fingers, perhaps adding an object to hold such as a feather, a long blade of grass or a flower.
- Play guess the gigantic toy by holding a small object close to the light source so its shadow looms large. This will work best indoors using a lamp or torch.
- Use small construction toys, such as wooden blocks or magnetic tiles, close to the light source to create huge towers on the screen. Your toddler can then knock them over and watch them tumble down!

Benefits for your toddler:

- Your toddler will be using their visual sense and sense of proprioception as they move their body and watch the resulting shadows.
- They will make discoveries about movement, light, patterns and shadows.

Building on:

- As you play outside or take a walk, point out the shadows that you can see, such as those made by trees, cars, the buggy or your own bodies.

> If using a lamp or torch as a light source, ensure it is placed safely where it cannot fall over and where your toddler can't reach any hot parts, such as the bulb. Ensure any wires are secured so as not to cause a trip hazard.

Skewers for chewers
A taste sensation

What you need:

A range of fruits, such as apples, oranges, kiwis and mangos

- A child-safe knife
- A chopping board
- Wooden skewers – snip the pointed end off with kitchen scissors
- A plate

The steps:

- Wash your hands together with your toddler.
- Introduce the fruits and engage your toddler in handling and smelling them. Draw their attention to details such as the shapes of the fruits, their colour, the texture of their skin, their weight and so on.
- Discuss with your toddler which fruits they prefer and which they are less keen on.
- Support your toddler to help you to peel the fruit (if necessary) and chop it into bite-sized pieces.
- Encourage your toddler to design a fruit kebab by threading the pieces of fruit onto the skewer, creating their own pattern.
- Ask your toddler to thread another kebab for a family member (who might prefer different fruits to them).
- Arrange your fruit kebabs on a plate ready to share with your family.

Benefits for your toddler:

- As they peel and chop, your toddler will be immersed in experiencing the range of fruits using all of their senses, in order to understand the appearance, texture, smell and taste of the fruits.

Building on:

- Encourage your child to alternate pieces of fruit to create a repeating pattern.

> ⚠ Always supervise your toddler when they are using a knife and while eating. Ensure the fruit is cut to a safe size to avoid a choking hazard.

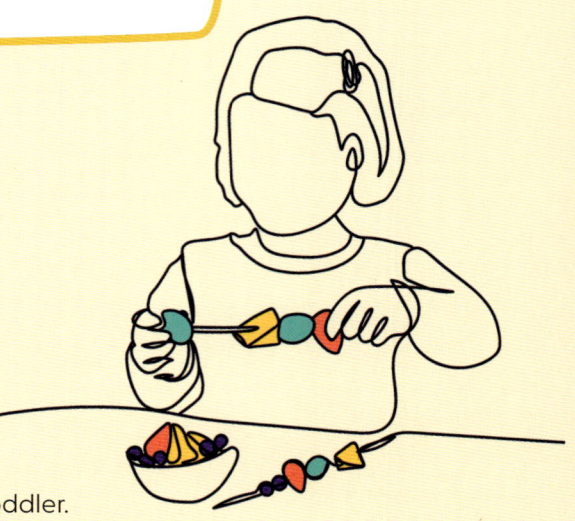

Hubble bubble toil and trouble
A simple and mobile potion kit

What you need:

- A natural outdoor area
- Recycled plastic pots
- Tools for grinding, mixing and stirring, such as a pestle and mortar, a tea strainer, spoons and wooden coffee stirrers
- A large jug or a bowl, made of plastic or metal
- A bottle of water (a recycled pump-action bottle works well)
- Tools for transferring mixtures, such as small jugs or funnels
- A small clear container, such as an empty jam jar

The steps:

- Set out to your chosen natural outdoor area. Together, forage for your potion ingredients – these might be petals, leaves, bark, soil, blackberries or elderflowers – your toddler might have many more ideas! Place each of your foraged items in the plastic pots.
- Discuss the environmental impact of your activity with your toddler and agree together how this could be reduced, for example, by gathering items that have fallen to the ground or by foraging in places where items are plentiful and there is enough left for wildlife to feed on.
- Return home and discuss potion possibilities and ideas – your toddler could make a gnome potion, a fairy perfume, a magic potion and so on. Let their imagination lead the way.
- Encourage your toddler to explore the range of tools to grind, mix and stir their potions.
- Use the funnel to decant the potion into a container to transport or store.

Benefits for your toddler:

- This activity involves all of the senses. Toddlers need lots of opportunity to use multiple senses together, in order to help to develop connections in their brain which support tasks that use multiple senses, such as hand–eye coordination.

Building on:

- Collect different aromatic plants, such as herbs or flower petals, to make pungent infusions.

> ⚠️ When foraging make sure you know what plants you are touching and ensure your toddler does not put them into their mouth. If you're unsure what a plant is, don't encourage your toddler to touch it. You can use a plant identifier app to learn more about plants.

Indoor obstacle course
Physical fun with furniture

What you need:

- Large removable cushions from a sofa or chair

The steps:

- Remove the cushions from your sofa or armchair and place them in a line on the floor with no gaps between them.
- Challenge your toddler to walk over the cushions. Can they also walk backwards over the cushions?
- After they have practised this, separate the cushions a little so that there are small gaps between each one. Challenge your toddler to step across from one cushion to the next.
- To increase the challenge even more, increase the gaps between the cushions again and demonstrate to your toddler how to jump with both feet from one cushion to the next.
- Allow your toddler to experiment with the heavy work of returning the cushions back to the sofa.

Benefits for your toddler:

- Your toddler will be challenging and developing their vestibular system as they move and regain balance on the unsteady surface.
- They will be receiving proprioceptive input as they travel in different ways and coordinate and sequence their movements.
- The heavy work of returning the cushions to the sofa also gives your toddler proprioceptive feedback.

Building on:

- If you have a smooth floor which allows you to pull a cushion along, you could see if your toddler can keep their balance sitting on the cushion whilst you slowly 'surf' them around the room.

> Test out the cushions on your floor before you play. On hard floors if the cushions slide around it won't be safe for your toddler to walk over them and we suggest you place the cushions on a carpet or rug instead.

Chapter 5

Language

Talking and listening

Language is of course impressive and it is such an exciting moment when your child says something that you can understand, but there are many other types of communication. For you and your baby, it started with something as simple as eye-contact and facial expression, and as they have grown into the toddler they are today – full of personality – they will have been using sounds, gestures, expressions and perhaps words to communicate. You are able to understand each other before your toddler masters spoken words, but sharing a common language certainly makes it easier.

You have been tuning into your toddler's early vocalisations, facial expressions and gestures since they were a baby. Your responses and actions to validate all of these communication attempts, no matter how tricky to decipher, will have encouraged your toddler to persevere to make their needs known. So it's a great time to congratulate yourself on the journey so far!

These forms of communication tell us so much – even as adults our body language continues to send powerful messages along with our words. Children don't start to talk until they first learn to understand words and what they represent – they will also need to closely watch the faces of adults and older children to see how to produce sounds through the coordination of the lips, teeth and tongue. In addition to this, children need to master the less visible and tricky elements of coordinating their vocal chords and breath to produce sounds.

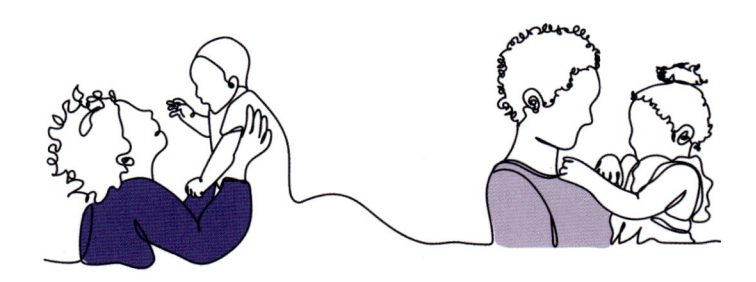

Plenty of talk and interaction together, during your everyday play and routines, provides wonderful opportunities for your toddler to hear language used in clear, repeated and predictable ways. Even though the talk may feel a little one-sided, each time you describe what you are doing or extend and elaborate on your toddler's early talk, they will have the opportunity to hear a wide variety of words and sentence structures within a familiar context. Lots of repetition of words in context and within the routine exchanges that we use throughout the day (Hello, how are you?) helps your toddler to understand the meaning of words and to link them to familiar objects or situations.

Once their first words are acquired your inquisitive toddler will be uplifted by the impact of having their words understood! This will drive their desire to communicate further.

> **Language allows social connection and the sharing of a culture.**
>
> Alistair Bryce-Clegg

Communication and language skills lay a foundation for other areas of development, guiding and supporting your toddler's thinking while underpinning their emerging literacy.

Tuning in, learning to listen and direct attention
The skills of tuning in, listening and paying attention will support your toddler to focus their attention and discriminate particular sounds from background noise. It's helpful to model good listening by looking at your toddler when they speak and following your toddler's lead as they direct your attention to a toy or an object. It is then possible to interact around this encounter by making follow-up comments, expanding and elaborating on what they say, or perhaps by asking questions. These situations, when two people are giving their attention to the same thing, are known as shared attention, and playfully engaging in these situations, for example by having a pretend cup of tea, is a wonderful way to hold your toddler's attention and to immerse them in language.

Learning and understanding new words

Word learning or vocabulary development involves your toddler learning to recognise and produce the sounds of words whilst also learning the meaning of those words. All the talk you direct to your toddler helps to scaffold the next step of development, and lots of this comes down to repetition of words in familiar routines and contexts.

You will subconsciously be thinking about how to help your toddler by adding just enough information to move their understanding on when you speak to them. This might be by moving from using one key word when you speak to your toddler, to starting to talk to them in short phrases with gestures and lots of repetition until they begin to understand the words. For example, if you used to say 'Train. Look train', then you will build on these phrases by adding new words to your toddler's replies, 'Yes, noisy train. Train going now'. Helping with pronunciation by repeating the words your toddler is struggling to pronounce correctly back to them in your reply, something called recasting, is often part of early conversations.

Early words are usually those with an emotional or social connection – words that are an important part of your toddler's daily experience. For example, if your household has a pet, your toddler may learn the words 'guinea pig', 'cat' or 'fish' early on. Names of close family members are also often attempted, along with the names of familiar, important objects (bottle, juice, car) or body parts (ear, eye, hair).

Your toddler will be able to move on to using decontextualised talk – which means referring to things and events not physically present in the 'here and now' but instead that might have happened in the past or in a story. This might include explanations of something that happened earlier in the day, talking during pretend play and talking about future events. Again, you can, and are most probably already (subconsciously) doing so, support these steps by adapting your language to make it just complicated enough for your toddler to learn from.

Decontextualised talk and imaginative play go together, not only for recreating real-world social situations from memory or experience but also for exploring fantastical possible worlds! Your toddler might not only mimic the appearance and behaviour of the shopkeeper, doctor or waiter, but also use their phrases and voices.

Early speech using combinations of words followed by more complex sentences

Gradually your toddler's repertoire of vocabulary will become more diverse and sophisticated. When children have learnt between 50 and 100 words, they often start to put these words together into short phrases.

They may delight in expressing needs or preferences such as a request for 'more milk' or a declaration of 'no coat!'. They may find it very satisfying that they can draw your attention to things of interest, saying, for example, 'look, bird!'. Your toddler will also understand your simple requests and instructions, such as 'show Grandad' or 'hold hands'. Along with these simple phrases, your toddler may also use a handful of familiar learned sequences (such as 'twinkle, twinkle, little star') or other phrases they hear often throughout the day.

Speaking confidently to adults and other children

Your toddler needs lots of opportunities to take part in conversations with people who care about them. Putting their own thoughts into words allows your toddler to express their preferences, interests and feelings verbally, although they may still combine these with plenty of gestures and expression for emphasis! Confidence will grow as their audience listens, responds positively and values their contributions.

Role of other cognitive developments on oral language

Interpretation of some complex sentences puts cognition to work too, as it requires the listener to hold information in their memory over time to work out the correct order of events. For example, 'Before you open the door, put your coat and wellies on'.

Oral language, reading and phonological awareness

Phonology is the set of sounds a language contains – think of them as the building blocks of talk. Reading is a really helpful way to expose your toddler to a whole range of phonemes, especially if you use different voices – for example, 'hissssssssing' the words of the snake or 'mooooooing' the words of the cow. Your toddler will begin to develop a good understanding of how sounds combine together to make up words as they explore the vocabulary, rhythm and rhyme within stories and songs. Books offer the opportunity to use more words in more complex sentences and to talk around the storyline.

Offering your toddler lots of opportunities to engage with books that fire their imagination and interest fosters a love of reading. It's beneficial to enable them to choose and look at books freely as well as to share them when read by an adult.

QR code

Don't forget to scan this QR code to find lots more child development content and bonus activity ideas from the team at My First Five Years.

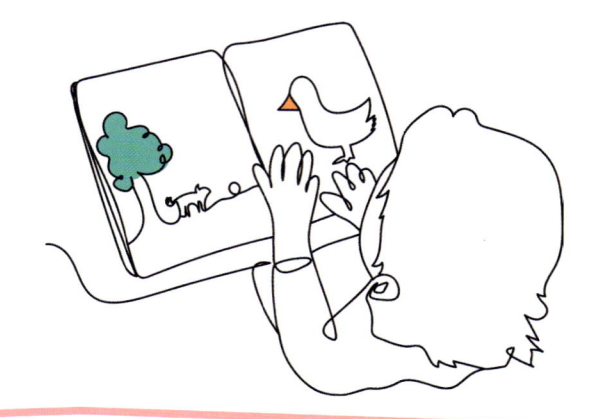

Shh! What can you hear?
A listening moment

What you need:

- A one-minute sand timer or a timer on a watch or smart phone

The steps:

- This activity can take place indoors or outdoors.

- Remind your toddler how good they are at listening and explain that you are both going to listen for one minute to all of the sounds that you can hear. It may be helpful to use the timer to illustrate the passing of the minute before you start the activity.

- Find a comfortable position, sitting or standing, and encourage your toddler to wiggle around and get comfortable ready to start the timer.

- Start the timer and model listening carefully to the environmental sounds that you can hear. If outside, you might listen to birdsong, traffic noise and the sound of the wind. If inside, you could listen to household sounds like appliances running, music playing, other people moving around or the weather against the window.

- When the minute has passed, discuss what sounds you both heard and what it was that made the sounds.

- If there are not many sounds that's okay as you can talk about how quiet and peaceful it is. It may also mean that you can hear your own breathing or the rustle of your own clothes as you adjust your position while listening.

Benefits for your toddler:

- Your toddler will be learning to channel their attention and to distinguish or pick out particular sounds from background noise.

Building on:

- When your toddler hears or recalls sounds, they may enjoy trying to reproduce a similar sound themselves. For example, the 'brmmm' of a car or the 'moo' of a cow.

- If your toddler hears a sound but doesn't know what might have made it, you can go on a 'noise hunt' to find out! Ask them to think about what kind of sound it was, if they have heard it before and perhaps which direction they think it came from, then let them lead you on a search around the area to see if you can track it down together.

What can it be?
Describing and recognising toys

What you need:

- A collection of your toddler's favourite small toy animals or pictures of animals
- A small bag or box

The steps:

- Start with a small selection of toy animals, this could be just two or three initially. Show the animals to your toddler and name each one. If they want to join in, you can ask your toddler to name the animals for you as you look at each one.
- Place the animals into the bag or box. Make sure you can either peek in to see what animal you will pull out next each time, or that you can feel the difference between them so you can describe each one in the next step.
- Describe a particular animal that you are going to pull out of the bag, but don't tell your toddler its name. For example, 'I'm choosing an animal that has a tail, horns and four legs'.
- Ask your toddler to guess the name of the animal. If your toddler finds it difficult to guess, you could help with more clues, perhaps describing the colour of the animal or the noise it makes.
- When your toddler gets the hang of the game, swap roles so that they can describe the animal for you to guess.

Benefits for your toddler:

- Your toddler will be expanding their vocabulary as they listen to and understand new descriptive words.
- Your toddler will develop the confidence to use their own descriptive language.

Building on:

- You could play this game with other collections or sets of toys. The toys could be based on transport – for example, cars, aeroplanes, buses and boats, or musical instruments – for example shakers, bells, small drums and whistles.
- This activity can be made more challenging by introducing a collection of household objects, such as items used for cooking or gardening. You could also describe the use of the item – for example, you might describe a spoon by saying, 'I use this to scoop up my cereal at breakfast'.

Let's get ready to go
Getting dressed

What you need:

- A selection of your toddler's clothes

The steps:

- Involve your toddler in finding and choosing the items of clothing they need for the day.

- Offer your toddler a couple of choices for each item of clothing as this provides an opportunity to talk about the similarities or differences between those items. You might say, for example, 'This top has short sleeves, but this one has long sleeves' or 'This woolly jumper is thick and warm. This cardigan is warm and has buttons'.

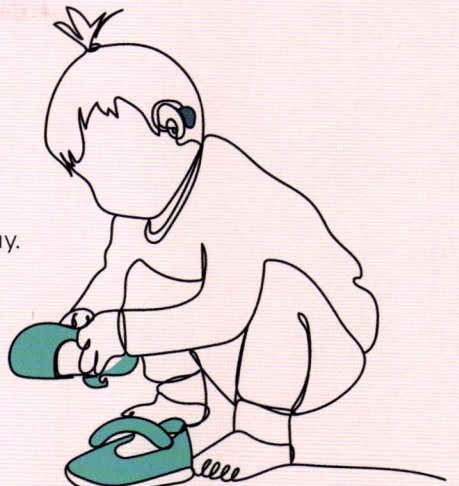

- As your toddler helps you to select each item of clothing, name it and talk through the process of putting it on, thinking about which body part it fits.

- If your toddler says something like, 'These shoes', you could expand on their words by replying, 'You want these red shoes'. Alternatively, if they say a single word, you could add to it and turn it into a short sentence.

- Continue to offer varied vocabulary by identifying fabric types, sizes of clothing and names of body parts, and by describing colours, patterns and details such as pockets, buttons, zips and collars.

Benefits for your toddler:

- Taking it slowly when getting ready to go out gives you plenty of time to chat and introduce your toddler to new words and their meanings in context. Expanding on your toddler's talk by repeating what they said with one extra detail or a more complete structure supports their language development.

Building on:

- Revisiting this activity and the associated vocabulary as part of your routine is helpful. You could revisit some of the language when your toddler gets undressed at bedtime.

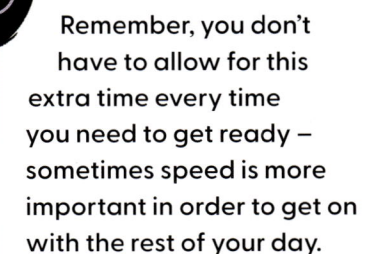

Remember, you don't have to allow for this extra time every time you need to get ready – sometimes speed is more important in order to get on with the rest of your day.

Open all hours
Setting up shop

What you need:

- Everyday items that you might buy in a shop, such as food, toys and books
- Real or imaginary money – this could be a pretend debit card and small box to 'beep' it on for payment
- A shopping bag

The steps:

- Set up your shop with your toddler – it can be as simple as setting items out on the floor or on a table. As you set up your shop, name and talk about the items that you will sell.
- Talk to your toddler about a recent trip to the shops, reminding them about where you went, who was there and what happened when you chose an item then paid for it. Tell them your new shop needs a customer and a staff member and let them choose who they would like to be first.
- If you are the customer, ask your child for an item that you would like, perhaps explaining why you need it. Try asking for two or three items at a time, encouraging your toddler to collect them.
- If you are the staff member, welcome your toddler to the shop and ask what they're looking for today. They might have a plan already or alternatively they may need you to prompt them to look at the items available if they are not sure.
- When playing, use phrases your toddler might hear in a real shop, such as 'Would you like a bag for this?', 'That will be £5 please, card or cash?', 'How much is this one?' and 'Thank you for your help!'.
- Swap roles so that your toddler has a turn at being both the customer and the member of staff.

Benefits for your toddler:

- Pretend play helps your child to build their understanding of the world and develop language to go along with the situation.
- When they are collecting several items, this supports their memory for listening to and following longer instructions.

Building on:

- Your toddler could make signs for their shop or labels for their items.

Next time you go shopping, give a short shopping list made of images to your toddler for them to help spot and shop for the things you need.

Library time
Sharing stories

What you need:

- A local library

The steps:

- Visit your local library with your toddler and register them for membership (this is free).
- Explore the children's section together – there will be board books, picture books, story books, information books and magazines.
- Ensure that you give your child plenty of time to browse and independently dip into the books that capture their interest, as well as sharing some stories together.
- Notice the type of books and magazines they are most interested in. These might be information books, lift-the-flap stories or stories about a particular character.
- Encourage your toddler to choose a few favourite books to borrow and take home.

Benefits for your toddler:

- Sharing books from an early age feeds your toddler's imagination, nurtures a love of reading and provides firm foundations for literacy.

Building on:

- Libraries also have stories, rhymes and songs on CDs that you might like to explore. Additionally, some libraries have story sacks with props that link to the story.

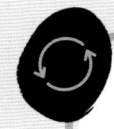

Many libraries have regular weekly sessions for babies and young children featuring stories, rhymes and songs. These are a great way to meet other parents and children.

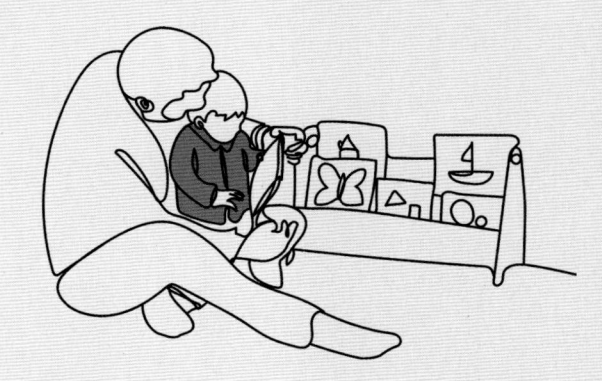

Ready, steady, go!
Traffic light game

What you need:

- A suitable space indoors or outdoors
- Green and red coloured paper or card (optional)

The steps:

- Explain to your toddler that red means stop and green means go – just like real traffic lights. If you are using coloured paper or card, hold these up to reinforce the words as you say them.
- The rules are that when you say green your toddler has to move, and when you say red they have to stop.
- When your toddler understands these rules, you could extend the game by introducing different ways of moving, such as running, spinning, crawling, dancing, jumping and rolling.
- Your toddler can then swap with you and have a turn at being in charge of the traffic lights!

Benefits for your toddler:

- This game helps your toddler to understand and follow simple instructions by using the words 'red' and 'green' to signal when to stop and go.
- If you say the words for the various actions as you do them, your toddler will begin to connect the meanings of these words with the actions.
- Your toddler will also be developing their concentration and listening skills as they pause and anticipate what comes next.

Building on:

- You could add an amber traffic light to signal moving on the spot – you might use this to represent 'get ready' and encourage your toddler to run on the spot when you say and show 'amber'.

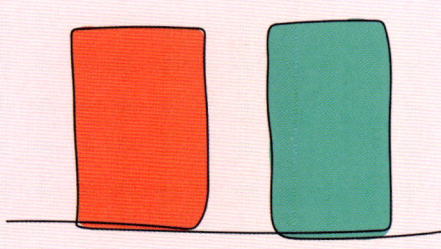

This is a great game to play with friends or family. You can challenge everyone to move at the same time or in a different way from the person next to them.

A trip to an unfamiliar shop
Exploring somewhere new

What you need:

- A few local shops to visit, such as a furniture shop, a DIY shop, a garden centre, a pet shop, a fabric shop and a charity shop

The steps:

- While you are on the journey to the shop, talk about what you can see, expanding on your toddler's comments. For example, you might say, 'Oh, I can see a bus over there, and people waiting to get on'. If your toddler adds, 'Dog!', you can expand on this saying something like, 'Oh yes, that little dog is waiting for the bus too'.

- You can also talk to your toddler about what they think they might see when they arrive. For example, 'We are going to arrive at the garden centre soon. There will be lots of plants and also lots of tools for gardening. You might see some spades – they will be bigger than your spade for the sand'.

- Explore the shop together, finding items that are new, unfamiliar or intriguing. Describe these things to your toddler naming them and focusing on details such as appearance (shape, colour, size and so on), function or – if relevant – their behaviour.

Benefits for your toddler:

- A trip to a new shop provides the opportunity to chat with your toddler about all of the novel and different things that can be seen there. Inviting your toddler to join in language-rich conversation will boost their understanding of words and how to use them.

Building on:

- Use this approach to add new vocabulary to your child's words at home, too. Talk about what you're making for lunch or what you're wearing, using lots of detail. For example, you could say, 'I'm wearing my red top. It's soft and warm'.

> Remember, things don't have to be very unusual or exciting to be new and interesting for your toddler – a change of shop or going to a different playground is all new for them!

Tell me more
Talking about experiences

What you need:

- Photos, objects and videos to prompt your toddler to talk about a recent experience you have shared together

The steps:

- Use your photos and other items as a prompt to inspire conversation. You can do this by having the photos or items out where both you and your toddler can see them, then starting to comment out loud about what you see or remember about them. You might point to one and say, 'This is us at the table. You have a balloon!'. Leave a pause for your toddler to share their thoughts and memories about the picture or item.

- Allow your toddler to take the lead in the conversation. This enables them to share the details of any experiences that are important to them. These might not be the obvious parts of the day!

- You can help your toddler to develop their storytelling skills by repeating and elaborating on their comments. For example, if you look at photographs of a trip to the park together, your toddler might comment, 'Park' or 'I go park'. You could then reply, 'Yes, we walked to the park'.

- If the photos are all of one day or trip, you could tell the story of the adventure in the order it happened by looking at the photos in turn. For example, 'First we had breakfast and you got crumbs in your hair, look! Oh, next we went on the bus. Here we are on the top waving to the camera'.

Benefits for your toddler:

- Recalling and sequencing past events orally is a great foundation for beginning to write, as your toddler will be practising organising and sequencing events. In order to write we need to be able to think about what word comes next and plan the order of our words and sentences. Although this comes naturally to adults, it is a skill that needs to be learnt over time. Any experiences of remembering and repeating a sequence of events will develop this skill.

Building on:

- When you are out and about with your toddler, photograph the small, but important, details they spot, such as a ladybird or a special leaf. Use these photos later when talking with your toddler to spark their enthusiasm.

Feeling the beat
Moving to the rhythm

What you need:
- A suitable space indoors or outdoors
- A selection of favourite music with different tempo and beat

The steps:
- Play music at home and have your own kitchen disco – jumping, swaying, marching and spinning!
- Once your toddler has had a chance to wiggle and dance freely, start showing them how you can match your movements to the beat of the song.
- Start with one simple movement to the beat, and when your toddler has got the hang of this, add in more actions or movements following a pattern.
- Try using a song or playlist that has a varying beat and tempo. When there is a change in the beat and/or tempo, explain to your toddler that you're changing your movements to match the new speed by moving faster or slower, or perhaps stopping when the music pauses.
- If your toddler is struggling to coordinate big movements with the beat of the song, try clapping along, patting a drum (or tabletop) or tapping a foot to the beat instead. This means your toddler will be able to focus more on the beat and less on keeping their balance as they move.

Benefits for your toddler:
- Your toddler will be refining listening and attention skills as they tune into and notice changes in the beat or tempo of the music, and will be able to match their movements to these.
- Identifying a beat in a piece of music involves your toddler separating and filtering out that sound from other sounds, which builds the skill of tuning into and segmenting the sounds within words.

Building on:
- If you have space in front of a mirror at home it's great for you and your toddler to check out your moves as you both follow the beat.

> When you are out for a walk you could march along together, singing a song or chanting a rhyme. If you can find two sticks you could tap out the beat as you march.

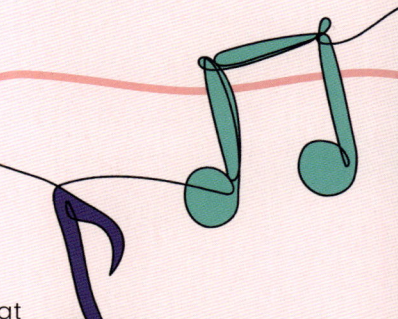

Tall tales
Making up stories

What you need:

- Characters for your story, such as play figures, soft toys, vehicles or animals
- A variety of fabrics to suggest story settings, such as green fabric for a forest, white fabric for a cold icy place and yellow fabric for a beach or desert
- Any other props from around the house to support your developing storyline

The steps:

- Explain to your toddler that you are going to make up your own story together.
- Ask your toddler to choose a favourite toy to be the main character.
- Help your toddler to think about the different parts of a story by asking them where the story will be set, such as at home, in a forest or in another place that is familiar to them. Use your fabric (or other props) to represent the setting of the story.
- Come up with ideas together about what might happen to your chosen character. Do they come up against a problem that they need to solve?
- Perhaps think about a real-life experience familiar to your toddler and weave this into your story, and involve members of your family as characters. You could also include elements of familiar stories you have read together.
- Act out the story together with the toy taking the lead, introducing some of your other characters as necessary.
- Retell the story and offer your toddler vocabulary and phrases to extend their ideas. For example, if they talk about there being snow, you can describe it using words like 'icy', 'crunching' or 'sparkling'. As they become more familiar with the story, encourage your toddler to add more detail by asking them about what the characters can feel, see, smell or hear.

Benefits for your toddler:

- Your toddler will see how to plan and sequence events within a story and, with your support, will learn how to put these events into words and sentences.
- Stories can help your toddler to make sense of their world as they voice their thoughts and feelings and explore events that might make them feel scared, anxious, excited or confused.

Building on:

- Take photos of the character(s) to help your toddler to sequence the events and retell the story to another family member.

Chapter 6

Cognitive

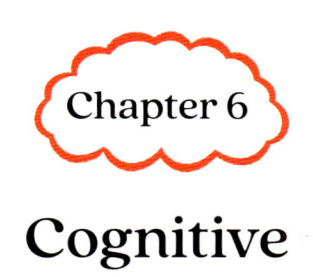

Making connections

Brain architecture is a term used to refer to all the connections made between neurons in the brain – there are billions of them! Babies' brains begin to develop before they are born, but there is a lot of development still to happen after birth. It's thought that toddlers are developing more than one million new connections between neurons per second, which might help you to understand why the world can seem so overwhelming to them at times.

New connections between neurons are formed when your toddler experiences something new, and are reinforced when that thing is repeated. This can be something such as a movement, a feeling in response to an event or a phrase being said.

Exploring the world and making connections between the things they experience involves cognitive development. Cognitive development refers to the process in which your child's brain gathers, processes and understands information. Receiving information from the senses is only the first stage of understanding; your child's brain will then try to make sense of this sensory stimulus, making connections between what their senses tell them and what they already know – for example, feeling something warm and recalling that hot things in the past have been dangerous to touch. Their brain may also make assumptions to overcome gaps in their knowledge, such as seeing a tall person with glasses and calling them 'Daddy' because they link the way their own dad looks and the way this person looks, and come to the conclusion that they must be referred to in the same way.

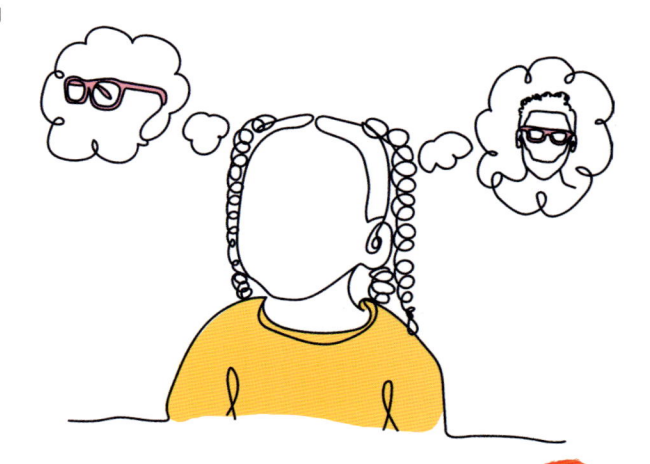

Developing new connections in the brain, and building up the cognitive skills to recall important details, will also help your toddler when they are receiving lots of information as it can allow them to decide what is 'salient'. In other words, filtering out what is most helpful and relevant and being able to ignore unnecessary information. At first your toddler has limited experience of filtering in this way and will not be able to decide how to maintain or switch their attention, so they might be easily distracted by a lovely noisy or shiny new toy, they may become upset by an unfamiliar loud noise, or they may find it hard to tune into your voice above background noise.

Gradually your toddler will begin to demonstrate a growing understanding of the world and culture that surrounds them. They will begin to understand their own role within this, both physically and socially, through experience and participation. For example, they may begin to understand social processes (such as how people greet each other or thank each other), how to join in with everyday activities (such as shopping or cooking) and what particular items and objects are used for (scissors for cutting, a comb for tidying hair).

Researchers believe that the first five years are a particularly important period for learning as it is a time when our brains are particularly plastic: this means our brain can change and adapt by building and strengthening connections and pruning away unused connections. This is a brilliant tool which prevents us from becoming overwhelmed by the number of connections and neural networks in our brain. It is also why repetition is so important for your toddler – the brain decides which connections to keep and which to prune away based on how frequently they're used.

Cognitive development is an essential part of overall development because it allows your toddler to build an internal model of the world that they can refer to. They will build a bank of past experiences and use these to predict what might happen when they encounter new situations or experiences, in this way connecting previous experiences with new learning.

Cause and effect

You may notice your toddler repeating actions over and over again, such as shaking an instrument, pushing a button, banging blocks together or dropping different objects. This repetition helps them to understand cause and effect – the idea that a specific action leads to a specific response. So, one object might bounce when they drop it but another object might smash.

Building up this bank of information through repetition and experimentation (including trying to repeat the action in ways that don't work) allows your toddler to use their knowledge to anticipate and make predictions about what might happen as a consequence of their own actions, or other people's actions, in different situations. This sense of the world being a predictable place helps your toddler not only to feel safe, but also to be able to adapt their actions and behaviour in ways that keep them safe, such as knowing that a cup of tea is hot and might cause pain or that a wet surface might be slippery and cause a fall.

Executive function and self-regulation

Executive functions are the cognitive skills which enable us to manage all the information being sent to our brain, and to use this information to make decisions that help us as we move through life. They enable us to focus our attention, prioritise tasks and needs, plan for the future and think flexibly enough to change those plans if needed. These same skills enable us to understand and manage our thoughts and emotions, and to control our impulses.

Your toddler's attention will initially be like a search light encompassing a wide area, but over time they will develop the ability to focus it to be more like a spotlight trained on a particular area of interest. Their brain will build the skills needed to filter distractions, prioritise tasks, set and achieve goals and control impulses.

Once your toddler has begun to master some executive function skills, they will begin to learn to use them to self-regulate. Self-regulation, or self-control, enables us to set and follow priorities and resist impulsive actions or responses. As these skills develop, your toddler will be able to understand and follow behaviour expectations and make healthy choices for themselves – for example, resisting eating all of the chocolate biscuits in one go!

As your toddler's working memory develops, they will be able to hold multiple pieces of information in their head over a short period of time. This allows them to follow simple instructions, such as 'Can you fetch your coat and then come back here?'. Working memory supports your toddler to know the sequence of steps in a familiar routine, such as getting dressed or washing hands, which allows them to become more independent.

Mind-minded talk

One way to support your toddler's cognitive development is through something known as 'mind-minded talk'. This is the process of talking through your thoughts out loud, giving your toddler a chance to hear and understand how the thinking process can work for others. Talking through your thought process, or narrating what your toddler may be thinking, also has the advantage of expanding the range of words you say to your child. For example, you might say, 'I have decided to put my coat on because it's raining outside'.

Symbolic play and representation

As they grow, your toddler will make the cognitive leap to enjoying symbolic play (using one object, or person, to represent another thing, such as using a block as a phone) and pretend play (using their imagination to develop symbolic play, such as by pretending to be someone else or giving thoughts and feelings to a toy).

You might see your toddler create storylines through pretend play, sometimes called role play, as they dress up and gather props to explore how it feels to be a shopkeeper or a bus driver. In order to pretend, your child needs to use their working memory to think about storylines and characters linking these to familiar situations or experiences and developing deeper understanding.

Your toddler will learn to maintain focus on their play or to stop and return to play if interrupted. They may plan, evaluate and change the storyline based on what happens around them or the actions of others involved in the play. Activities that foster creative play and social connection teach your toddler how to negotiate with others and, over time, provide opportunities for directing their own actions with decreasing adult supervision.

Your toddler may demonstrate their understanding of representation, or symbolism, through symbolic play. So, for example, a doll might represent a real baby, a stick could become a magic wand or a wooden block might be a bar of chocolate. Symbolic play is a stepping stone to literacy and numeracy. When we write letters and numbers, we're using symbols for what we want to convey.

Symbolic mark-making

An understanding of symbolism will support your toddler's developing awareness that marks can be used symbolically to carry meaning, such as a cross to indicate a kiss in a card or a set of marks to represent the letters of their name. This understanding will support your toddler's journey to becoming a writer because word learning is symbolic.

Early mark-making often occurs spontaneously in play, where the purpose and the meaning of representation are within your toddler's control. You might notice your toddler writing a list during role play, or creating a sign, label or menu for their restaurant, or even making a tally to represent quantity.

QR code

Don't forget to scan this QR code to find lots more child development content and bonus activity ideas from the team at My First Five Years.

Make a favourite sandwich
Tell others how to do it!

What you need:

- Two of slices of bread
- Butter or spread
- A few favourite sandwich fillers, such as cheese, cucumber and tomato
- A child-friendly knife
- A cheese grater (optional)
- A chopping board
- A plate
- A smart phone or a camera to take photos

The steps:

- Help your toddler to take a photo of each of their chosen ingredients, describing and naming each one and discussing their appearance, smell and taste. Take a photo of your toddler completing each of the steps of the activity.
- Support your toddler to butter both pieces of bread and then ask them which ingredient they would like to add next.
- Encourage them to add each ingredient one at a time, supporting them to chop, cut or grate.
- Emphasise that the last step is to put the second slice of bread on top of the sandwich filling.
- Look at the photos of the activity together and talk about what happened at each step.

Benefits for your toddler:

- Your toddler will experience planning and sequencing the steps needed to complete a simple task. Explaining these steps to others helps them to remember the sequence.

Building on:

- Your toddler could make a sandwich for a family member or friend; encourage your toddler to explain how they made it when they present it to the person.

Always supervise your toddler while they are making and eating food, and ensure they only have access to equipment that is safe for them to use.

I wonder what might happen next
Anticipating events in familiar stories

What you need:

- A favourite storybook that your toddler knows well

The steps:

- Settle down somewhere comfortable to read together.
- Encourage your toddler to hold the book and turn the pages.
- Begin to read the story, but pause frequently so that your toddler can fill in words or repeated refrains.
- As your toddler turns the page comment, 'I wonder what will happen next...' giving your toddler plenty of time to answer.
- You might notice your toddler likes to read favourite stories over and over again. A familiar story can make your toddler feel safe as they know it stays constant and predictable when other things in their life are changeable.

Benefits for your toddler:

- Your toddler's familiarity with the story will help them to sequence the main events and predict what is coming next. This gives them a sense of ownership of the story.
- Over time experiencing the beginning, middle and end of various stories helps your toddler to understand how events are sequenced.

Building on:

- You could create a small box of favourite books and encourage your toddler to 'read' these to other family members or even their toys. They might make up their own versions using the pictures, or remember lots of key moments from the story and retell these – either way, they are building on their knowledge of sequences.

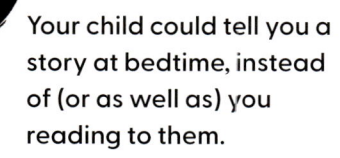

> Your child could tell you a story at bedtime, instead of (or as well as) you reading to them.

What's missing?
A memory game

What you need:

• A tray

• A selection of six familiar household objects, such as a spoon, a small toy, a shoe, a sock, a TV remote control, a set of keys and a crayon

• A piece of fabric to cover the tray, such as a tea towel or a pillow case

The steps:

• Show your toddler the selection of objects. Name them as you look together and talk about what they look like and what they do.

• Place three objects on the tray and let your toddler have a close look.

• Cover the tray with the fabric and ask your toddler to close their eyes.

• Secretly remove one of the objects and hide it behind your back.

• Ask your toddler to open their eyes, remove the fabric and see if they can identify which object is missing.

• If they find this easy you could increase the number of objects on the tray.

Benefits for your toddler:

• Your toddler will be challenging their working memory by trying to remember all of the objects on the tray.

• This activity also helps them to develop their attention and focus on a task.

Building on:

• After a couple of turns, change roles and let your toddler remove an item whilst your eyes are closed.

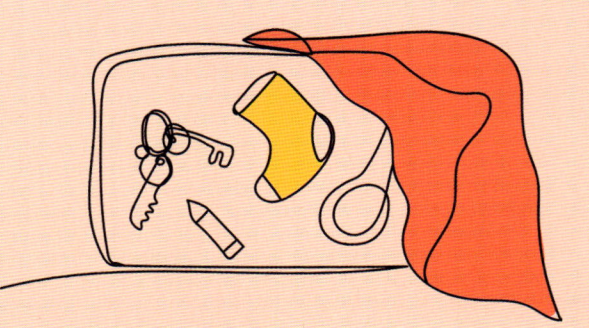

If your toddler enjoys this game, it can be played while out and about. It's ideal to play at the table of a café or restaurant using cutlery, toys and a napkin while you wait for your food to arrive.

Recreate a familiar place
Open-ended role play

What you need:

- A variety of clothing and accessories, such as hats, belts, bags and scarves
- A large cardboard box

The steps:

- Offer the selection of clothing and accessories and the box to your toddler and notice how they begin to play. They might dress up as a particular character or pretend to be in a familiar place that they have visited. The box might be used as a vehicle, shop counter, dog bed or simply a good place to collect treasures. Your toddler's imagination can turn a simple box into whatever they need for their game!

- If they seem stuck for ideas, you could suggest role playing a situation that you know interests them or that they have experienced recently, such as visiting a shop, a train station or a restaurant – assure them that they can create anything they want to.

- Follow your child's lead in the play, supporting them by finding additional props that fit their pretend play, such as a few pots and pans for a café, and taking the role of other characters.

Benefits for your toddler:

- Your toddler is using their memory of familiar situations, experiences and the people involved in these in order to recreate them in their play.

- Pretend play allows your toddler to revisit and explore familiar situations from the perspective of the characters, therefore developing deeper understanding of the fact that other people might have different thoughts and needs to them.

- Your toddler will need to think flexibly as they respond to others who are participating in the play.

Building on:

- You might like to expand your toddler's collection of props for pretend play by visiting local charity shops or asking family and friends for items that are no longer needed.

- As your toddler returns to themes in their play they may develop a storyline, and over time their play can become more complex through repetition.

- Inviting friends to join play can support your toddler to begin to explain and negotiate their own ideas and to respond to the thoughts and ideas of others.

Brick play
Stacking, bridging, enclosing and representing

What you need:
- A selection of wooden bricks
- A floor space large enough to sit together and build

The steps:
- Encourage your toddler to begin to build with the bricks and notice how they play.
- They might begin by stacking the bricks horizontally and vertically, or they might begin bridging between bricks – they may even begin to create simple enclosures.
- Allow them to explore freely and copy the kind of play they are exploring, perhaps by making similar structures or helping them to place their bricks.
- Talk to your toddler as they play in order to describe what they are doing. This could include language of size (big, small, tall, wide), language of shape (square, rectangle) or language of position (under, on top, behind, next to).

Benefits for your toddler:
- Your toddler will be planning and sequencing their actions and maintaining focus to complete their goal.
- They may be comparing the sizes and shapes of the blocks and selecting the most suitable for their task.
- Your toddler may begin to explore simple maths. For example, counting the blocks or considering distance when they are lining them up or bridging gaps.

Building on:
- Over time, your toddler might make patterns and explore symmetry, or make simple structures to represent objects, buildings or places they know.
- You could add natural objects for your toddler to construct with, such as stones, branches and logs.

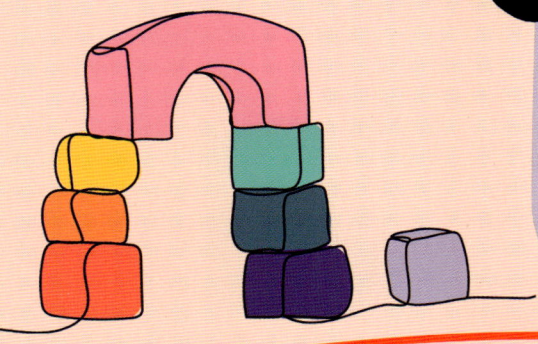

> You can use this same approach when your child is playing with other toys – or even when doing simple tasks like getting dressed – by talking about the size, shape and position of what they're doing.

An amazing soundscape
Make your own musical story

What you need:

- A range of instruments that can be used to make a musical story, such as:
    * A set of bells or a bunch of keys to show something magical
    * An empty plastic or glass bottle to blow on to represent the wind
    * A drum or an upside-down saucepan and spoon to indicate a dramatic change
    * A pair of shells for a galloping horse
    * Small stones in a tin to represent something rattling

The steps:

- Explore the kinds of sounds the instruments or objects make. Encourage your toddler to close their eyes as they listen and decide what the noises remind them of.
- You might find that your toddler wants to move in response to the sounds, pretending to be blown by the wind or marching to the drumbeat and so on. Join them in their actions.
- After lots of free exploration, you could weave some of the sounds into a simple story, creating a storyline around the sounds and using them to add atmosphere to suggest different events, landscapes or weathers.

Benefits for your toddler:

- Your toddler will be encouraged to participate in planning and sequencing the story using the sounds as a prompt for ideas, and so will begin to view themselves as a storyteller.

Building on:

- Retell a familiar story from a book using your instruments to enhance particular parts of the story.
- Draw simple symbols to represent each instrument and stick each symbol to an individual piece of card. You could then organise the cards in different sequences to make your own musical score.

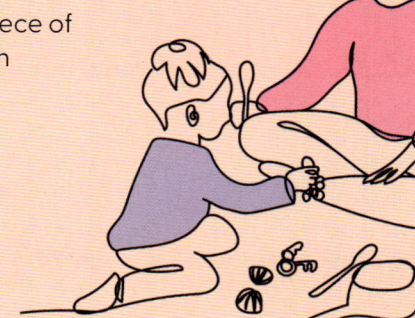

Full to the top
Exploring capacity in the bath

What you need:

- A home-made water play kit including items such as:
    - ✶ Bowls or plastic tubs of different sizes
    - ✶ Measuring scoops or spoons
    - ✶ Small empty bottles, such as food colouring bottles, shampoo bottles or children's drinks bottles
    - ✶ Larger plastic bottles, such as milk bottles

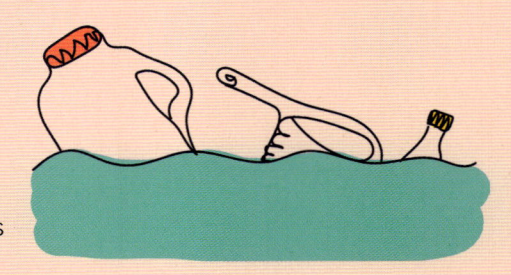

The steps:

- Fill the bath for bath time and add the items from the water play kit.
- Give your toddler plenty of time to investigate filling, emptying and transferring water from one container to another.
- Comment on their play, noticing when a container is full, empty, half full or overflowing.
- Your toddler might also notice the larger containers becoming heavier as they get full, or floating on top of the water when they are empty.

Benefits for your toddler:

- Your toddler will be exploring concepts such as capacity, floating and sinking, in a hands-on way, along with beginning to understand some of the associated language.
- Having a play kit available to use regularly at bath time helps your toddler to return to their investigations, to check the same thing happens each time and to extend their explorations.

Building on:

- As you watch your toddler play, take note of those items they are most interested in and use this information to extend the range of containers in the kit.

> ⚠ Always supervise your toddler around water, and ensure the water temperature is safe and suitable before they play.

A pictorial calendar
What's happening this week?

What you need:
- A large piece of paper
- A pen
- A ruler
- Colouring pencils

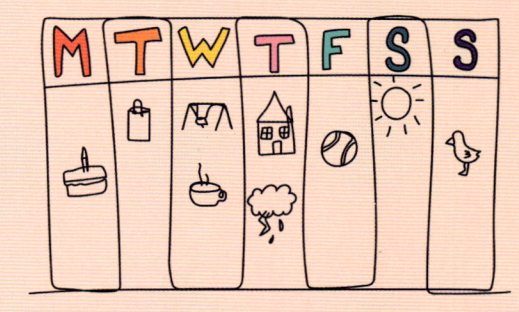

The steps:
- Draw a weekly calendar on your paper, talking to your toddler about how you need to divide the paper into seven columns, ready to label each column with the name of the day of the week.
- Talk about the sequence of the days of the week as you label the columns, asking your toddler to think about what day it is today, what day it was yesterday and what day it will be tomorrow.
- Suggest to your toddler that they could draw a picture on the calendar to show something that happened in the past on a previous day of the week. Do not worry if the picture is not recognisable – you could add a symbol or a couple of words underneath their drawing for clarity.
- Ask them to also draw a picture or symbol to represent something that is planned to happen on a future day that week.
- Put the calendar up somewhere at your toddler's height so that they can refer to it and add to it during the week.

Benefits for your toddler:
- Marking the passing of time helps your toddler to begin to develop a clearer understanding of the concept of time in a personal sense – for example, breakfast time, bedtime and storytime. A sense of time is gained gradually during the process of living through timespans.
- This activity helps your toddler to explore vocabulary related to time, such as before, after, next and tomorrow, along with the names of the days of the week.

Building on:
- Devise consistent symbols for reoccurring events, such as birthdays (perhaps a cake) or toddler groups that you attend. You could use your toddler's drawings for the symbols.

You could use a simple calendar to record other household routines, such as ticking whether the dog or cat has been fed!

Let's go shopping
Noticing signs and logos

What you need:

- A smart phone or a camera to take photos (optional)

The steps:

- Whilst you are out and about, draw your toddler's attention to the different signs and logos that you spot. These might be signs and symbols for shops, brand logos, street signs or car badges.
- Notice any that your toddler seems particularly interested in and perhaps take a photo.
- When you return home, you could draw or print out some of the signs or logos for you and your toddler to talk about together. Chat about what they look like and where you spotted them.
- Your toddler could use the signs and logos in their play. For example, you could copy the logo for the supermarket you usually go to and stick it on a wooden block so that your toddler's toy cars can drive to the supermarket.
- Next time you and your toddler go out, see if you can both spot the logos that you have drawn or photographed.

Benefits for your toddler:

- Your toddler will be learning that marks can be used symbolically to carry meaning. This understanding will support your toddler's journey to becoming a writer because word learning is symbolic.

Building on:

- Over time, your toddler could build a collection of favourite logos. These could be stuck onto small cards to be used for a spotting game when on a longer journey or when with friends.
- Your toddler might like to try drawing the logos themselves, or they could pick out the colours for you when you are drawing together.

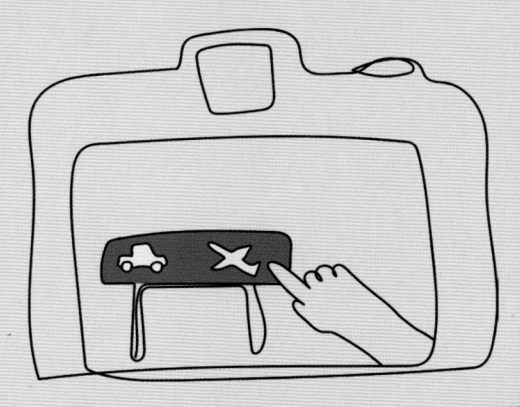

Mix and match
Can you find the other sock?

What you need:

- Some (clean!) socks belonging to your family

The steps:

- Choose a selection of socks of different sizes, colours and patterns.
- Gather the socks together in a heap – perhaps starting with three or four pairs so that the task doesn't feel too overwhelming.
- Encourage your toddler to help you to sort the socks into their matching pairs. Talk aloud as you do this, modelling your thinking. For example, 'I've got this sock with red stripes, it's a big one, so I'm looking for another big one with stripes'. Pause and see if your toddler can find the missing sock!

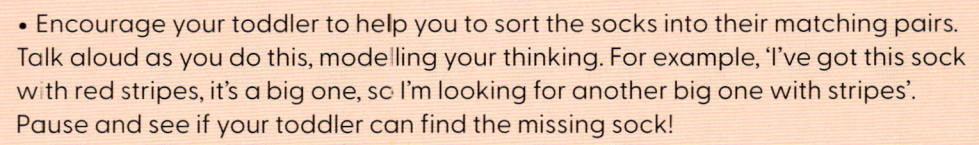

Benefits for your toddler:

- Your toddler will be developing their ability to focus on a task or thought in order to make the match and will be having to hold multiple pieces of information in their head as they do this, developing their memory skills.
- Your toddler will also be getting a chance to test their ideas about similarities and differences as they find the matching socks.

Building on:

- You can gradually increase the number of pairs of socks in the pile which will increase the complexity of the task for your toddler, meaning they will need a longer attention span to complete it.
- Your toddler could then help you to identify who the socks belong to and help you return them to the correct drawer in the house.

> Playing games like this can help involve your toddler in some of the tasks that need to be done around your home, which will help them understand what tasks they can help with as they get older.

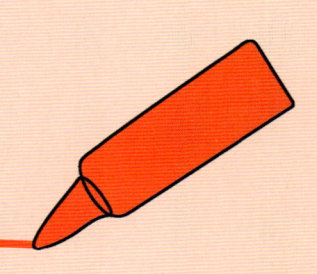